Practice Single Best Answer Questions for the Final FRCA

A Revision Guide

Practice Single Best Answer Questions for the Final FRCA

A Revision Guide

Edited by

Hozefa Ebrahim
Specialist Registrar, Queen Elizabeth Hospital, Birmingham,
Associate Clinical Teaching Fellow,
University Hospitals Birmingham, UK

Khalid Hasan
Consultant and College Tutor,
Queen Elizabeth Hospital, Birmingham, UK

Mark Tindall
Consultant and College Tutor,
Russells Hall Hospital, Birmingham, UK

Michael Clarke
Specialist Registrar, Queen Elizabeth Hospital, Birmingham,
and Advanced Pain Fellow, University of Birmingham, UK

Natish Bindal
Consultant in the Department of Anaesthesia,
and Consultant, Queen Elizabeth Hospital, Birmingham, UK

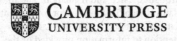
CAMBRIDGE
UNIVERSITY PRESS

CAMBRIDGE
UNIVERSITY PRESS

University Printing House, Cambridge CB2 8BS, United Kingdom

One Liberty Plaza, 20th Floor, New York, NY 10006, USA

477 Williamstown Road, Port Melbourne, VIC 3207, Australia

4843/24, 2nd Floor, Ansari Road, Daryaganj, Delhi - 110002, India

79 Anson Road, #06-04/06, Singapore 079906

Cambridge University Press is part of the University of Cambridge.

It furthers the University's mission by disseminating knowledge in the pursuit of education, learning and research at the highest international levels of excellence.

www.cambridge.org
Information on this title: www.cambridge.org/9781107679924

© Cambridge University Press 2013

First published 2013

A catalogue record for this publication is available from the British Library

Library of Congress Cataloging in Publication data
Practice single best answer questions for the final FRCA : a revision
guide / edited by Hozefa Ebrahim . . . [et al.].
    p. ;   cm.
Includes bibliographical references and index.
ISBN 978-1-107-67992-4 (pbk.)
I. Ebrahim, Hozefa.
[DNLM: 1. Anesthesia – methods – Examination Questions.
2. Anesthesia – adverse effects – Examination Questions. WO 218.2]
617.9´6076–dc23

                                                        2012013424

ISBN 978-1-107-67992-4 Paperback

....

Contents

Principal contributors

Edward Copley
Specialist Registrar in Anaesthesia
West Midlands Deanery, Birmingham, UK

Anna Pierson
Specialist Registrar in Anaesthesia
West Midlands Deanery, Birmingham, UK

Richard Pierson
Specialist Registrar in Anaesthesia
West Midlands Deanery, Birmingham, UK

Contributors

Michael Allan
Specialist Registrar in Anaesthesia
West Midlands Deanery, Birmingham, UK

Natish Bindal
Consultant Anaesthetist
Queen Elizabeth Hospital, Birmingham, UK

Catriona Bentley
Specialist Registrar in Anaesthesia
West Midlands Deanery, Birmingham, UK

Hannah Church
Consultant Anaesthetist
Queen Elizabeth Hospital,
Birmingham, UK

Michael B Clarke
Advanced Pain Trainee
Specialist Registrar in Anaesthesia
West Midlands Deanery,
Birmingham, UK

Lloyd Craker
Consultant Anaesthetist
North Staffordshire Hospital, UK

Nicholas Crombie
Consultant Anaesthetist
Queen Elizabeth Hospital,
Birmingham, UK

Neil H Crooks
Specialist Registrar in Anaesthesia and
Intensive Care Medicine
West Midlands Deanery,
Birmingham, UK

Hozefa Ebrahim
Specialist Registrar in Anaesthesia and
Intensive Care Medicine
West Midlands Deanery,
Birmingham, UK

Ian Ewington
Specialist Registrar in Anaesthesia
and Intensive Care Medicine
West Midlands Deanery,
Birmingham, UK

James Geoghegan
Consultant Anaesthetist
Queen Elizabeth Hospital,
Birmingham, UK

Au-Chyun Nicole Goh
Clinical Fellow in Paediatric Intensive
Care Medicine
Birmingham Children's Hospital, UK

Andrew G Haldane
Specialist Registrar in Anaesthesia
West Midlands Deanery, Birmingham, UK

Khalid Hasan
Consultant Anaesthetist and College Tutor
Queen Elizabeth Hospital, Birmingham, UK

Max Simon Hodges
Specialist Registrar in Anaesthesia
West Midlands Deanery, Birmingham, UK

Eric Hodgson
Chief Specialist Anaesthesiologist,
Inkosi Albert Luthui Central Hospital
Honorary Senior Lecturer,
Nelson R Mandela School of Medicine,
Durban, South Africa

Asim Iqbal
Clinical Fellow in Hepatobiliary Anaesthesia
Specialist Registrar in Anaesthesia
West Midlands Deanery, Birmingham, UK

Paul Jeanrenaud
Consultant in Intensive Care Medicine and
Anaesthesia
Whiston Hospital, Merseyside, UK

Emily Johnson
Specialist Registrar in Anaesthesia
West Midlands Deanery,
Birmingham, UK

Deepak Joseph
Specialist Registrar in Anaesthesia
West Midlands Deanery,
Birmingham, UK

Michael McAlindon
Specialist Registrar in Anaesthesia and
Intensive Care Medicine
West Midlands Deanery,
Birmingham, UK

Craig McGrath
Consultant Anaesthetist
Queen Elizabeth Hospital, Birmingham, UK

Randeep Mullhi
Specialist Registrar in Anaesthesia and
Intensive Care Medicine
West Midlands Deanery, Birmingham, UK

Rebecca Paris
Specialist Registrar in Anaesthesia
West Midlands Deanery, Birmingham, UK

Sachin Rastogi
Pain Fellow
The Hospital for Sick Children,
Toronto, Canada

Simon Smart
Consultant Anaesthetist
Queen Elizabeth Hospital,
Birmingham, UK

Insiya Susnerwalla
Specialty Trainee in Anaesthesia
North Western Deanery, Manchester, UK

Alifia Tameem
Specialist Registrar in Anaesthesia
West Midlands Deanery, Birmingham, UK

Mark Tindall
Consultant Anaesthetist
Russells Hall Hospital, Dudley, UK

Laura Tulloch
Specialist Registrar in Anaesthesia and
Intensive Care Medicine
West Midlands Deanery,
Birmingham, UK

Abbreviations

AAA	abdominal aortic aneurysm
AChR	acetylcholine receptor
ACT	activated clotting time
ACTH	adrenocorticotrophic hormone
ADH	antidiuretic hormone
AIR	anaesthesia-related rhabdomyolysis
AKI	acute kidney injury
ALSG	advanced life support group
ALI	acute lung injury
APTT	activated partial thromboplastin time
ARDS	acute respiratory distress syndrome
ARF	acute renal failure
BMI	body mass index
BMS	bare metal stent
BP	blood pressure
CABG	coronary artery bypass graft
CAS	central anticholinergic syndrome
CDH	congenital diaphragmatic hernia
CDI	*Clostridium difficile* infection
CK	creatine kinase
CMRO$_2$	cerebral metabolic oxygen replacement
CNB	central neuraxial block
CNS	central nervous system
CO	cardiac output
COHb	carboxyhaemoglobin
CPB	cardiopulmonary bypass
CPP	chronic pelvic pain
CPSP	chronic postsurgical pain
CRF	chronic renal failure
CRPS	complex regional pain syndrome
CSE	combined spinal–epidural
CSF	cerebrospinal fluid
CT	computerized tomography
CTPA	computerized tomography pulmonary angiogram
CRT	cardiac resynchronization therapy
CSWS	cerebral salt-wasting syndrome
CXR	chest X-ray
DAPT	dual antiplatelet therapy
DES	drug-eluting stent
DI	diabetes insipidus
DLT	double lumen tube
DKA	diabetic ketoacidosis

DMD	Duchenne's muscular dystrophy
DMSO	dimethyl sulphoxide
DVT	deep vein thrombosis
ECMO	extracorporeal membrane oxygenation
ECT	electroconvulsive therapy
EPO	erythropoietin
ERCP	endoscopic retrograde cholangiopancreatography
ETT	endotracheal tube
EVAR	endovascular aortic aneurysm repair
EVLWI	extravascular lung water index
FEV$_1$	forced expiratory volume in 1 second
FES	fat embolism syndrome
FFP	fresh frozen plasma
GA	general anaesthetic
GABA	gamma amino-butyric acid
GBS	Guillain–Barré syndrome
GCS	Glasgow coma score
GFR	glomerular filtration rate
GI	gastrointestinal
HCAI	healthcare-associated infection
HDU	high-dependency unit
HFOV	high-frequency oscillatory ventilation
HITT	heparin-induced thrombotic thrombocytopenia
HLHS	hypoplastic left heart syndrome
HR	heart rate
IABP	intra-aortic balloon pump
IBW	ideal body weight
ICDSC	intensive care delirium screening checklist
ICP	intracranial pressure
ICS	intraoperative cell salvage
ICU	intensive care unit
ID	internal diameter
INR	international normalized ratio
LBBB	left bundle branch block
LBW	lean body weight
LMA	laryngeal mask airway
LMWH	low molecular weight heparin
LRTI	lower respiratory tract infection
LV	left ventricle
MAC	minimum alveolar concentration
MAOI	monoamine oxidase inhibitor
MELD	model for end-stage liver disease
MEN	multiple endocrine neoplasia
MG	myasthenia gravis
MPM	mortality prediction model
MR	magnetic resonance

MRI	magnetic resonance imaging
MVR	mitral valve replacement
NCA	nurse-controlled analgesia
NIBP	non-invasive blood pressure
NPV	negative predictive value
NSAID	non-steroidal anti-inflammatory drug
OLV	one-lung ventilation
OSA	obstructive sleep apnoea
PA	pulmonary artery
PAC	pulmonary artery catheter
PAFC	pulmonary artery flotation catheter
PCA	patient-controlled analgesia
PCI	percutaneous coronary intervention
PD	Parkinson's disease
PDPH	postdural puncture headache
PEEP	positive end-expiratory pressure
PICU	paediatric intensive care unit
POCD	postoperative cognitive dysfunction
PONV	postoperative nausea and vomiting
PPH	postpartum haemorrhage
PPV	positive predictive value
PRIS	propofol-related infusion syndrome
PT	prothrombin time
PTC	post-tetanic count
PTE	pulmonary thromboembolism
PVL-SA	Panton–Valentine leukocidin-producing *Staphylococcus aureus*
RA	right atrium
RASS	Richmond Agitation Sedation Score
RSI	rapid sequence induction
RV	right ventricle
SAH	subarachnoid haemorrhage
SAPS	simplified acute physiology score
SBE	subacute bacterial endocarditis
SIADH	syndrome of inappropriate antidiuretic hormone
SJW	St John's wort
SNRI	serotonin and noradrenaline reuptake inhibitor
SSRI	selective serotonin reuptake inhibitor
SUNCT	short-lasting, unilateral neuralgiform headache
TACO	transfusion-associated circulatory overload
TAP	transversus abdominis plane
TBI	traumatic brain injury
TBSA	total body surface area
TBW	total body weight
TCA	tricyclic antidepressant
TCI	target-controlled infusion
TEG	thrombo-elastograph

TENS	transcutaneous electrical nerve stimulation
TIVA	total intravenous anaesthesia
TLS	tumour lysis syndrome
TMJ	temporomandibular joint
TOE	transoesophageal echocardiogram
TOF	train of four
TRALI	transfusion-related acute lung injury
TSH	thyroid stimulating hormone
TTE	transthoracic echocardiogram
UFH	unfractionated heparin
URTI	upper respiratory tract infection
vCJD	variant Creutzfeldt–Jakob disease
VAE	venous air embolism
VC	vital capacity
VF	ventricular fibrillation
VT	ventricular tachycardia
VTE	venous thromboembolism
vWF	von Willebrand's factor
WP	widespread pain index

Classification of questions by topic

Category					
Basic sciences	A23, B9	D2, D22	F16 K15		H22
Cardiac and thoracic anaesthesia and intensive care medicine	D25 B3, B4, B13, B20	E2, E8, E9, E10, E13	F7, F21 A28, C24	G28	H5, H7, H9 J25, J28
Burns and trauma	A12, B25	K3, K11			
Equipment and clinical measurement	D1, D5			G30	
General anaesthetic practice	A2, A3, A4, A5, A6, A25, A26, A27, A30	C2, C3, C4, C21, C26, C28, C29, C30, C1	F12, F18, F20, F22, F23, F25, F26, F28, F29, F30	G2, G3, G4, G17, G21, G23, G26, G27, G29	H4, H8, H11, H16, H26
	B11, B12, B14, B15, B18	E1, E3, E4, E6, E7, E11, E30	J2, J12, J13, J16, J17, J18, J22, J29, J30		K1, K16, K21, K24, K25, K27, K29, K30
	D3, D4, D25, D27, D28, D30				
Intensive care medicine	C5, C9, C13, C17, C7, C12, C15, C27, E24	D6, D14, D15, A1, A7, A9, A10, A11, A17, A19, A29, B1, B2, B5, B6, B7, B22, B26, B28, B30	F1, F4, F9	G5, G8, G11, G12, G13, G25	H1, H12, H17, H30
			J3, J7, J11, J23, J26		K2, K6, K9, K10, K14, K17, K24, K25
Liver anaesthesia and medicine	E19	F11	G14, G16	H18, K17, K21	J18

Category					
Neuro-anaesthesia and intensive care medicine		E28		H10, H14, H25, H28	J5, J8
Obstetric anaesthesia	D19, D23 A20, A24 B8, B17, C18, C22	E14, E18	F17 J4, J19, J27	G18, G20, G22	H2, H6, H19 K18, K22, K26
Paediatric anaesthesia and intensive care medicine	D12, D16, D20, D24 A13, A16, A21 B16, B24 C10, C14, C19, C23	E12, E17, E21, E26, E27	F5, F13, F14	G6, G9, J9, J14, J20, J24	H3, H15, H20, H24 K7, K12, K19, K23, K28
Acute and chronic pain management	D9, D13, D17, D21 A14, A18, A22 B10, B19, B27 C8, C11, C16, C20	E5, E15, E16, E20, E25	F3, F6, F10, F15, F19	G7, G10, G15 J1, J6, J10, J14, J15, J21	H21, H23, H27 K8, K13, K20
Regional anaesthesia	D7 A8, B23, B29, C6, C25	E29	F2, F8	G19, G24	H29, K4, K5
Trauma and orthopaedics	D10, D11, D26	E23		G1	H13
Transplant surgery	D18	E22			
Vascular anaesthesia	D29		F24, F27		

Foreword

Since man has existed there has been a basic, innate human drive to help the sick and, whenever possible, to return them to health. Superimposed on this constancy of intent has been a steady and progressive improvement in the ways of managing illness. Anaesthesia and its related specialties of intensive care medicine and pain management have been instrumental in allowing these developments to occur. In so doing they too have had to meet and overcome new problems. These range from those posed by rapid recovery case anaesthesia via safer childbirth to the management of increasingly complex patients with reduced physiological reserves.

Through its Charter, the Royal College of Anaesthetists has a public responsibility to ensure that this clinical progress is not only maintained, but also that the knowledge to achieve it is both taught and examined. It is to the credit of the specialty that for many years it has led the way in preparing trainees and fellows for the task ahead. Over time, the College examinations have undergone huge changes: the ones I sat in the late 1970s were very different from those of today. Throughout, however, the college has maintained a constant theme of making the examinations fit for purpose in the context of current and future practice. Whilst frustrating the many who have had to cope with this change, the effect has been of enormous public benefit.

This book has been produced in response to the recent variation of educational strategy in the Final Examination: the introduction of the scenario-based single best answer question. For me its publication is welcome on two grounds. Firstly, there is no doubt it will help those preparing for the examination: the coverage goes across the whole syllabus, the clinical settings are relevant and it encourages learning based in the reality of the clinical environment. Secondly, it is a book generated and completed by the energy of young anaesthetists, both trainees and consultants. With such enthusiasm in the ranks, the future of the specialty looks bright.

I wish the book, its authors and all those who read it the very best of luck for the future.

Peter Hutton PhD, FRCA, FRCP, FInst Mech E, Consultant Anaesthetist and Hon Professor, UHB FT and University of Birmingham

Foreword

The requirement by the General Medical Council that assessments of specialist competence include reliable tests of knowledge has secured the position of multiple choice examinations as an essential component in postgraduate specialist examinations. The challenge for those creating MCQs and for candidates taking the examination is that this device does not readily permit expression of the nuances and complexities of everyday medical practice. The thinking that underpins the construction of MCQs and the 'correct answer' is therefore of considerable importance. This compendium of single best answer questions intended as revision for the FRCA examination achieves this task admirably by providing detailed answers to each set of questions, which were themselves derived from, and refined by, experienced senior anaesthetists as well as by those in training. The questions are broad-ranging, and are relevant to intensive care medicine as well as to the confines of the operating theatre. They are also a valuable educational resource for tutorials, and a tool for continuing professional development.

Julian Bion FRCP, FRCA, FICM, MD Professor of Intensive Care Medicine, and Dean of the UK Faculty of Intensive Care Medicine, Queen Elizabeth Hospital, University of Birmingham

Introduction: angle of attack

Over the years, the FRCA examination has steadily evolved with many incremental changes that have resulted in a progressively more modern and fair test of knowledge. It has always been a rigorous examination in terms of depth and breadth, setting a high standard. The examination is embedded into the curriculum, with the primary and final being prerequisites for accessing intermediate and higher specialist training, respectively.

The oral examinations have moved towards a much more structured examination, where there is a pre-planned amount of material to cover. This has resulted in a more consistent examination that has greater validity and reliability. The wording and material of the MCQ examination have been continually updated to contain clearer and more concise language; older questions are continually modernized and occasionally removed from the college bank. Many mourn the loss of the negatively marked MCQ; however, this has all been to make the examination process fairer and more transparent.

The latest change to the Primary and Final FRCA is the introduction of the single best answer question. In the examination, 30 MCQ questions have been replaced by 30 Single Best Answer (SBA) questions.

The reason to use this book when preparing for the Final FRCA is that we believe this book offers the most realistic 'Final FRCA' experience. All the questions in this book have been written by practising anaesthetists with an interest in education and examination preparation. Each of these questions has then been carefully reviewed to ensure it is of the appropriate level for the FRCA and relevant to the syllabus.

The questions in this book have the appearance, construct and feel of a FRCA question. Unlike MCQs, there is a paucity of college questions in the public domain. This book will give the most life-like experience of the actual examination.

The MCQ can be used as a good test of knowledge, with a high degree of validity and reliability. However, this type of question can only test a small area of factual recall. It is more difficult to test understanding or application of that knowledge.

The SBA, however, allows for a deeper question that can require application of knowledge from a number of areas to allow the deduction of the correct answer. A realistic scenario can be created and varied in many ways, with multiple correct options then presented. It is up to the candidate then to select the best response.

When referring to Miller's triangle of clinical performance, multiple true–false (MTF) questions test the 'knows' and the properly constructed SBA will test the candidate's 'know how' and also 'show' level. It does this by allowing the setting of a scenario that may entail integrating knowledge from several domains and applying them to arrive at a best response.

In the SBA question all the responses will be correct; however, one will be the 'single best' response. This needs to be borne in mind when tackling such a question, and hence a good grounding with knowledge and clinical judgement is vital.

This type of question is already in use in undergraduate examinations and by the GMC in the assessment of poorly performing doctors. They also have a key role in overseas examinations such as FANZCA and US board examinations. An increasing number of UK-based examinations are incorporating these questions into their tests.

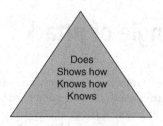

Let's examine the anatomy of the SBA question.

Firstly, there will be a description setting a scenario. It will contain all the vital information required to answer the question. This is not designed to mislead, or trick the candidate.

Secondly, there will be a question. The types of question are: What is the next most important treatment? What would you do next? Ideally, the question will ask a 'what next?' type rather than a negative response such as 'which is least likely?'.

Thirdly, in the FRCA SBA there are five responses. The candidate must choose the single best option. Currently, this is scored with four marks for a correct response and zero for an incorrect response.

If one were to draw a hypothetical line with incorrect options at one end and correct options at the other, then all the options will be at the 'correct' end of the line. Choosing the single best will require integrating knowledge and the use of clinical judgement.

The approach to answering the question should be structured to have the highest likelihood of success when choosing the answer. The incorrect options are termed distractors, and that perfectly describes their function.

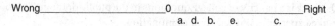

Here option c. represents the best response.

If one imagines a hypothetical line that one 'sees' after a question: the responses can be placed on a line where 0 is neither right nor wrong with a 'wrong' end of the line and a 'right' end of the line. The answers in a SBA will not be wrong (as a statement in themselves), but could be wrong in the context of a question. Much more likely is that the responses will ALL be correct responses, but one will be better than the others.

The challenge is to pick the 'single best answer'. This type of question is designed to reward the knowledgeable candidate. Hence there is no substitute for gaining a good base knowledge. Beyond this, certain approaches will help to identify the correct response quickly.

The cover up

Initially, when reading the scenario, cover the answers. Read the scenario carefully and then read the question. Without revealing the options, think about the best answer to that question.

Once you have done that, uncover the options. If what you thought is in that list, then that is the answer. Mark it and move on.

Discount the unlikely

If your answer is not amongst the options, then read all the options. You now need to start discounting the less likely options. It will help to re-read the scenario and question; then examine the options.

The easiest to discount will be statements that are untrue. A well-written SBA will try to avoid having this; nonetheless, some questions may have these and it should be straightforward for an informed candidate to discount them.

Protocols and guidelines make good material on which to base SBA questions. Often, the options will have distractors that contain elements that help with rejecting the incorrect responses, for example, an odd drug or dosing, incorrect next step or escalation of treatment. It is in these types of scenario that one needs to be familiar with standard UK practice.

Narrow the odds

Very occasionally even the most well-read candidate will come across a question that may be difficult to answer. In such situations a best guess may be needed. The chance of getting the correct answer can be improved by reducing the number of responses to guess from. There are often one or two options that may be relatively easily discounted, leaving one to guess from a pool of 2–3 statements rather than 5.

As in MCQ questions, look for statements such as 'always' or 'never'; or similar strong elements. These responses are rarely correct.

If one cannot narrow any of the options, then leave the question and move onto the rest of the paper. One may come across another question or a piece of information that helps you either to find the answer, or to narrow the options.

Ultimately, there is no substitute for a good background knowledge, based on strong basic science. In my experience the candidates who seem to struggle the most are those who, in their preparation for the FRCA, retreat completely into studying, neglecting the real clinical world where much of our knowledge is reinforced by clinical practice.

One's reading should include the RCOA's CEPD journal that accompanies the BJA. This is not just a rich source of quality information about the science and practice of anaesthesia, but is also a first port of call for examiners looking for inspiration to formulate questions for the FRCA. Likewise, protocols such as ALS, ATLS, BTS (asthma), ARDSnet and NICE provide rich sources for question writers.

After doing all the required reading and preparation, one must practise doing these types of question before sitting the exam for real. This book will offer the most realistic simulation of the SBA component to the correct standard in the Final FRCA.

Good luck, and study to aim for a first-time pass.

Khalid Hasan

Acknowledgements

We gratefully acknowledge Ed Copley, Richard Pierson, Anna Pierson and all the authors who contributed towards this book. Thank you for accommodating our constant requests for changes and improvements, and our many deadlines along the journey. It has been a pleasure working with you all.

A special thank you goes to Emily Johnson and Professor Peter Hutton for their advice on manoeuvring around the complex world of medical publications.

We express our sincere appreciation to Mrs Durriyah Ebrahim for her painstaking review of the entire manuscript; and all the recommendations for developments with grammar and layout.

Most of all, we must also thank our better halves; Tasneem, Tehseen, Charlotte and Marie for their patience and support during the writing of this book, and their ongoing encouragement for all our literary endeavours.

HE

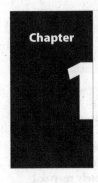

Chapter

1

Paper A – Questions

A1

A 40-year-old female who is intubated and ventilated following a subarachnoid haemorrhage (SAH) 7 days previously has a serum sodium concentration of 128 mmol/l and serum osmolality of 270 mOsm/kg.

Which of the following statements is true?
a. Cerebral salt-wasting syndrome (CSWS) is rarely associated with SAH
b. Cerebral salt-wasting syndrome is associated with a reduced serum osmolality
c. To diagnose SIADH, the patient must be clinically dehydrated
d. SIADH almost always requires pharmacological treatment
e. To diagnose SIADH urine osmolality must be greater than serum osmolality

A2

An 82-year-old female undergoes total hip replacement under general anaesthesia. She receives an intravenous induction and volatile maintenance, with propofol and isoflurane, respectively. In recovery she becomes extremely agitated and appears to be hallucinating, in association with a sinus tachycardia at a rate of 110 bpm.

Which of the following drugs, if administered during the procedure, is most likely to be responsible for her current clinical state?
a. Atropine 0.6 mg
b. Morphine 5 mg
c. Ephedrine 6 mg
d. Isoflurane 1.1%
e. Cyclizine 50 mg

A3

The commonest source of airborne micro-particles in the operating theatre is:
a. Staff failing to wear facemasks
b. Foot traffic into and out of theatre
c. Staff wearing home-laundered theatre clothing
d. Intraoperative use of a forced air warmer (e.g. *Bair Hugger®*)
e. Staff failing to wear footwear covers

Practice Single Best Answer Questions for the Final FRCA, ed. Hozefa Ebrahim, Khalid Hasan, Mark Tindall, Michael Clarke and Natish Bindal. Published by Cambridge University Press. © Cambridge University Press 2013.

A4

The introduction of the agent Suggamadex has drastically changed the management of aminosteroid-induced neuromuscular blockade.

Which of the following facts concerning its use is most accurate?

a. It can be used to rapidly reverse blockade induced by vecuronium, rocuronium and pancuronium
b. A deep block, characterized by no train of four (TOF) twitches, but a post-tetanic count (PTC) of 1–2 can be successfully reversed using a dose of 2 mg/kg
c. If rocuronium is used in a dose of 1.2 mg/kg for a RSI, it can be completely reversed after 3 minutes using a dose of 12 mg/kg
d. The activity of the oral contraceptive pill may be reduced by Suggamadex
e. The speed of reversal of neuromuscular blockade is slower if a volatile anaesthetic has been used to maintain anaesthesia

A5

Anaesthesia provided for electroconvulsive therapy (ECT) is frequently provided in remote locations and the conduct of anaesthesia may influence the efficacy of treatment.

Which of the following statements is most correct?

a. It is recommended that anaesthesia must be provided by a consultant anaesthetist
b. The presence of an anaesthetic machine is mandatory
c. Pipeline oxygen must be available
d. Propofol should be avoided as it prevents the induction of an adequate seizure
e. Suxamethonium is used primarily to prevent musculoskeletal injury

A6

The provision of general anaesthesia in the MRI scanner has many equipment considerations.

Which of the following statements is most accurate?

a. Equipment designated as magnetic resonance (MR) safe will function normally and not interfere with the correct operation of the MR imaging equipment
b. MR compatible equipment should pose no safety threat to either patients or staff
c. MR conditional equipment has been shown to demonstrate no known hazards in a specified MR environment
d. 3-tesla (T) MRI scanners are quicker, more efficient and cause fewer problems with monitoring than 1.5-T scanners
e. The use of temperature probes should be avoided

A7

A 62-year-old male admitted to the ICU following emergency repair of ruptured abdominal aortic aneurysm repair has developed multisystem organ failure and thrombocytopenia. He is prescribed continuous haemofiltration with an ultrafiltrate of 35 ml/kg per hour. The lifespan of the filter is short due to problems attributed to clot formation despite using unfractionated heparin. You have just been informed that the patient has heparin-induced thrombotic thrombocytopenia.

What first-line strategy would you employ to improve the lifespan of the filter?
a. Change the unfractionated heparin to LMWH
b. Prescribe warfarin to maintain INR 1.5–2.5
c. Use epoprostenol instead of heparin
d. Administer the replacement fluid pre-filter
e. Administer danaparoid

A8

Analgesia for upper limb procedures can be provided by means of a brachial plexus block. For operations on the proximal part of the upper limb, a relatively high approach is required and an interscalene block is used.

Which of the following is true?
a. Diaphragmatic paralysis occurs commonly after bilateral stellate ganglion block
b. An interscalene block commonly misses the roots of the ulnar nerve
c. There is significant risk of intrathecal injection at this level
d. 2% of interscalene blocks result in recurrent laryngeal nerve palsy
e. 60% of interscalene blocks result in a phrenic nerve block

A9

A 27-year-old man on the ICU underwent decompressive craniectomy 7 days following an acute subdural haematoma. He remains intubated and ventilated and has become agitated with a heart rate of 120 bpm and a BP of 80/40 mmHg. His urine output is 200 ml/h. Further serum and urinalysis reveals the following results:

| Serum | osmolality 300 mOsm/l; | Na^+ 120 mmol/l |
| Urine | osmolality 300 mOsm/l; | Na^+ 40 mEq/l |

Which of the following would be the most appropriate next step in your management?
a. Fluid restriction
b. Fluid resuscitation with 0.9% NaCl
c. Demeclocycline
d. Fludrocortisone
e. Desmopressin

A10

A patient with a known history of migraine presents to the emergency department with a severe migraine, which has failed to respond to his usual treatment of paracetamol and ibuprofen.

Which of the following is most likely to help him with his acute pain?
a. Sumitriptan
b. Amitriptyline
c. Codeine
d. Propanolol
e. Pizotifen

3

A11

A 19-year-old female presents to the emergency department stating that she took an overdose of 50×500 milligram paracetamol tablets 30 minutes ago. It is decided to attempt gastrointestinal decontamination.

Which of the following regimens would be the most appropriate in order to reduce paracetamol absorption in this patient?
a. 30 millilitres of ipecacuanha administered by mouth to induce vomiting
b. Whole bowel irrigation with 1.5 litres/hour polyethylene glycol via nasogastric tube until the effluent runs clear
c. Whole bowel irrigation with 2 litres/hour polyethylene glycol via nasogastric tube until the effluent runs clear
d. Gastric lavage via a 30 F orogastric tube
e. Activated charcoal 50 grams administered by mouth

A12

A 26-year-old male weighing 70 kg has presented to the emergency department following a house fire. He is estimated to have full thickness burns to the chest, abdomen, back and right arm. He has partial thickness burns to the right leg.

Using the Parkland formula, you estimate that the amount of replacement fluid the patient requires in the first 8 hours is:
a. 8820 ml Hartmann's solution
b. 8820 ml 4.5% human serum albumin solution
c. 6300 ml Hartmann's solution
d. 6300 ml 4.5% human serum albumin solution
e. 17640 ml Hartmann's solution

A13

An understanding of hypoplastic left heart syndrome (HLHS) can aid understanding of the fetal heart, and can demonstrate how ventilatory strategies can be used to manipulate physiology.

Which statement is correct regarding HLHS?
a. It is the most frequently occurring duct-dependent cardiac malformation, and may initially be managed with a prostaglandin infusion to maintain duct patency and systemic circulation, until the child reaches 3 kg in weight
b. Children should have S_pO_2 in the normal, or near normal range following repair in the neonatal period (Norwood procedure)
c. If the S_pO_2 is 88% following Norwood procedure, a sensible first option would be to decrease the F_iO_2
d. Rising lactate and hypotension following initial surgery can be an indication to start vasopressors
e. Patients with a Fontan circulation benefit from a low circulating volume as this offloads the single ventricle, and reduces cardiac work

A14

Fibromyalgia is part of a spectrum of chronic pain disorders. Progress has been made in the treatment of chronic pain, but reliable long-term treatment is still problematic.

In the treatment of fibromyalgia, which of the following is most correct?
a. Tricyclic antidepressants reduce pain by increasing 5-HT release
b. SSRIs improve mood but have little effect on pain
c. MAOIs have no role in chronic pain
d. Lidocaine infusions of 5–8 mg/kg over 2 hours reduce daily pain scores
e. The 'Magill' scale describes patient responses to TENS therapy

A15

Intra-aortic balloon pump (IABP) increases the oxygen delivery to the myocardium and decreases the myocardial oxygen demand thereby improving its function, especially in heart failure.

Which of the following physiological effects are not seen with a well-functioning IABP?
a. ↑ Aortic diastolic pressure
b. ↓ Left ventricle end-diastolic pressure
c. ↑ Coronary blood flow
d. ↓ Renal blood flow
e. ↓ Haemoglobin levels by up to 5%

A16

A 12-year-old boy with moderate learning difficulties requires multiple dental extractions due to poor dentition and previous dental abscesses. He has multiple previous admissions to hospital. He is crying, appears terrified and is refusing to have topical local anaesthetic cream applied or to co-operate.

What is the best initial approach to this child?
a. Decline to anaesthetize the child on this occasion until he is calm
b. Manually restrain him in the anaesthetic room with the consent of his carers, and attempt a gas induction
c. Manually restrain the child on the ward to give parenteral sedation
d. Offer oral midazolam, starting at 0.1 mg/kg, with a maximum dose of 15 mg. If that does not work, re-book the case for another day
e. Offer oral midazolam, starting at 0.1 mg/kg, with maximum dose of 15 mg. Repeat the dose if the first does not work

A17

Pleural effusions are caused by a number of pathologies.

Which of the following statements regarding pleural effusions is true:
a. The pH of normal pleural fluid is 7.2
b. Congestive heart failure is a common cause of an exudative pleural effusion
c. Liver cirrhosis can cause an transudative pleural effusion
d. A transudative pleural effusion is characterized by a protein content of >30 g/l
e. According to Light's criteria, an exudative pleural effusion has a pleural fluid/serum LDH ratio of <0.6

A18

A 75-year-old patient with type 2 diabetes had a below-knee amputation under a combined spinal–epidural block. Three months later he is still complaining of phantom limb pain despite simple analgesics.

Which treatment has the best evidence to support its use in this scenario?
a. Mirror-box therapy
b. Oxycodone
c. Spinal cord stimulation
d. Ketamine
e. Gabapentin

A19

A 75-year-old female who is being treated with broad-spectrum antibiotics for ventilator-associated pneumonia develops abdominal distension and diarrhoea. Her white cell count is 20×10^9 and her temperature is 38.9 °C. You suspect that she has *Clostridium difficile* infection.

The most appropriate first-line treatment would be:
a. enteral vancomycin 125 mg qds
b. enteral metronidazole 400 mg tds
c. intravenous metronidazole 400 mg tds
d. enteral vancomycin 125 mg qds and intravenous metronidazole 500 mg tds
e. enteral vancomycin 500 mg qds

A20

After the 2007 CEMACH report, the Royal College of Obstetricians and Gynaecologists published guidance on thromboprophylaxis during pregnancy.
In which of the following clinical scenarios should thromboprophylaxis be continued for at least 7 days postnatally?
a. Age >35
b. Obesity (BMI >30)
c. Patient requiring antenatal thromboprophylaxis
d. Previous venous thromboembolism
e. Caesarean section in labour

A21

A 10-year-old boy with appendicitis has been listed for an urgent appendicectomy. He has some mild learning disabilities and is on sodium valproate for his epilepsy. His seizures are generally well controlled but his mum reports that his last grand-mal seizure was 2 days ago.

In anaesthetizing the child with epilepsy, which of the following is true?
a. Regional blockade or local anaesthetic infiltration should be avoided, since local anaesthetic toxicity can present with tonic–clonic seizures
b. Sevoflurane is preferable to isoflurane for maintenance of anaesthesia
c. Fentanyl is a preferable opioid to alfentanil
d. Atracurium infusion is preferable to rocuronium boluses since higher doses of neuromuscular blockers are required
e. Pethidine is a preferable opioid to morphine

A22

A 60-year-old man is referred to your pain management clinic via his GP. He gives a 6-month history of worsening lumbar back pain that is not eased with rest or simple analgesics. He suffers from ulcerative colitis, which is well controlled with mesalazine. On examination, he has a good range of lumbar spine movement, normal power and reflexes but reduced sensation in the L5 dermatome on the right.

What would be the next step in his management?
a. Arrange a lumbar epidural
b. Prescribe a strong opioid and review in 3 months
c. Refer for a neurological opinion
d. Refer for a course of physiotherapy
e. Request an MRI scan

A23

Pharmacokinetics of anaesthetic drugs in the morbidly obese patient changes significantly. Which of the following statements with regard to anaesthetic drug dosing in the morbidly obese is true?
a. Thiopentone sodium dose for induction is calculated according to total body weight
b. The dose of suxamethonium is calculated on the basis of lean body weight
c. The dose of hyperbaric bupivacaine 0.5% for subarachnoid block should be halved
d. Rocuronium dose depends on total body weight
e. Propofol used as infusion for total intravenous anaesthesia should be based upon total body weight

A24

Haemorrhage is one of the top five most common causes of maternal death according to the 2010 CMACE report.

Which of the following is correct regarding blood transfusion in the pregnant state?
a. Red cell alloimmunization is most likely to occur in the second trimester
b. Only Kell-negative blood should be used for transfusion in women of child-bearing age
c. Massive blood loss may be defined as the loss of one blood volume within a 24-hour period
d. Anti-D prophylaxis is required if a Rh D negative woman receives Rh D positive FFP or cryoprecipitate
e. The platelet count should not be allowed to fall below $75 \times 10^9/l$ in the acutely bleeding patient

A25

Cardiac resynchronization therapy (CRT) has a role to play in the management of patients.

It is indicated for:
a. Moderate aortic stenosis
b. Paroxysmal atrial fibrillation
c. Recurrent ventricular tachycardia
d. Restrictive cardiomyopathy
e. LBBB

A26

Postoperative cognitive dysfunction (POCD) is increasingly recognized as a cause of post-operative morbidity.

With regard to its predisposing factors, which of the following statements is true?
a. There appears to be a genetic predisposition
b. Early POCD is more likely in patients with lower levels of education
c. Prolonged POCD is associated with significant periods of intraoperative hypoxaemia
d. Prolonged POCD is associated with increased duration of anaesthesia
e. Prolonged POCD affects 1% of patients of more than 60 years of age after major surgery

A27

Diabetes is the most common endocrine disorder affecting UK patients. It is a complex disorder and can have multi-systemic effects, many of which are relevant to anaesthetic practice.

When managing these patients, which is the greatest consideration?
a. Polydipsia results from a direct effect of increased plasma glucose concentration on the supraoptic nucleus
b. Patients with autonomic neuropathy have increased variability of their heart rate on inspiration as they are unable to increase their stroke volume
c. Regional blocks are useful in diabetic patients, and adrenaline should be used to increase the duration of block
d. Pain in diabetic patients may increase insulin requirements by as much as 20%
e. Undiagnosed infections are present in 4% of diabetic patients

A28

A broncho-pleural fistula is an abnormal communication or a passage between the bronchial tree and the pleural space, causing a persistent leak.

If these patients are mechanically ventilated, the management strategy should be:
a. Low tidal volumes and high respiratory rate
b. Reduced inspiratory pressures
c. High tidal volumes and low respiratory rate
d. Low inspiratory times and high PEEP
e. High inspiratory times and low PEEP

A29

You are asked to review a 68-year-old woman with shortness of breath and hypotension on the surgical HDU, 24 hours after an anterior resection for bowel cancer.

Which of the following statements regarding venous thromboembolism (VTE) in this patient is most true?
a. In high-risk patients D-Dimer tests should be taken before subjecting patients to the radiation load of a CTPA
b. Around 25% of PTE present with haemodynamic instability
c. Caval filters may increase rates of VTE

d. A high D-dimer result is highly suggestive of PTE
e. Patients with suspected PTE should be treated with anticoagulants immediately even if no imaging is available

A30

Which is the most important consideration that should be observed when performing laser airway surgery with an endotracheal tube (ETT) in place:

a. Inspired oxygen concentration should be kept as low as possible
b. Nitrous oxide may help maintain a low F_iO_2, which will help avoid airway burns
c. Saline-soaked gauze or pledgets should be placed around the ETT, to eliminate the risk of ignition
d. The ETT cuff should be filled with a mixture of methylene blue and saline, to dissipate heat and make cuff rupture obvious
e. Efficient smoke evacuation is mandatory near the operating site to protect the surgeon from smoke plumes

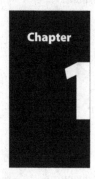

Paper A – Answers

A1

Answer: e.

The diagnostic criteria for SIADH are:

- Hypotonic hyponatraemia (serum sodium < 135 mmol/l and serum osmolality < 280 mOsm/l)
- Urine osmolality > serum osmolality
- Urine sodium concentration > 18 mmol/l
- Normal thyroid, adrenal and renal function
- Clinical euvolaemia

SIADH is often a self-limiting disease.

Cerebral salt-wasting syndrome (CSWS) is characterized by renal loss of sodium resulting in polyuria, natriuresis, hyponatraemia and hypovolaemia. It is the clinical signs of dehydration that differentiate it from SIADH. CSWS is predominantly associated with SAH and traumatic brain injury. The biochemical criteria for CSWS are:

- Low or normal serum sodium
- High or normal serum osmolality
- High or normal urine osmolality
- Increased haematocrit, urea, bicarbonate and albumin as a consequence of hypovolaemia

Bradshaw K, Smith M. Disorders of sodium balance after brain injury. *Contin Educ Anaesth Crit Care Pain* 2008; **8**(4): 129–133

A2

Answer: a.

This patient is most likely to be suffering from the *central anticholinergic syndrome (CAS)*. This is a disorder caused by cerebral penetration of antimuscarinic drugs, leading to a syndrome of central excitation or depression. It may thus be characterized by emergence delirium and agitation or by reduced consciousness level and coma.

CAS is frequently associated with peripheral anticholinergic side effects including dry mouth, tachycardia, blurred vision and urinary retention. Any anticholinergic drug able to

Practice Single Best Answer Questions for the Final FRCA, ed. Hozefa Ebrahim, Khalid Hasan, Mark Tindall, Michael Clarke and Natish Bindal. Published by Cambridge University Press. © Cambridge University Press 2013.

cross the blood–brain barrier may be implicated, including atropine and hyoscine. Other candidate drugs include antihistamines, antipsychotics, and tricyclic antidepressants, some of which demonstrate anticholinergic activity.

The diagnosis and treatment of CAS may be assisted by the anticholinesterase drug physostigmine, though symptoms may recur after its effect ceases.

Nair VP, Hunter JM. Anticholinesterases and anticholinergic drugs. *Contin Educ Anaesth Crit Care Pain* 2004; **4**: 164–168.

Sinclair RCF, Faleiro RJ. Delayed recovery of consciousness after anaesthesia. *Contin Educ Anaesth Crit Care Pain* 2006; **6**: 114–118.

A3

Answer: b.

This question illustrates an important point with respect to infection control. Facemasks are only required for staff within the sterile surgical field. Home laundering of theatre clothing is acceptable as long as the clothing is not worn outside theatre. Forced air warmers that are appropriately maintained provide filtered air without particles. Footwear covers do not reduce particles, but reliably contaminate the hands of those using them! Traffic through the theatre is the most significant source of microparticles and should be minimized, particularly while the incision is open.

American Society of Anesthesiologists Task Force on Infectious Complications Associated with Neuraxial Techniques (2010). Practice advisory for the prevention, diagnosis, and management of infectious complications associated with neuraxial techniques. *Anesthesiology*; **112**: 530–545.

A4

Answer: d.

Suggamadex is a gamma-cyclodextrin molecule that is indicated for the rapid reversal of aminosteroid-induced neuromuscular blockade. It is effective when rocuronium or vecuronium have been used (but not pancuronium), the speed of action being slightly slower with vecuronium. Its rapid and complete reversal of rocuronium-induced blockade may provide a viable alternative to the use of suxamethonium. It works by binding the neuromuscular blocker directly and therefore has minimal side effects.

Several dose-finding studies have been performed, and the recommended doses for use are as follows:

- For reversal of shallow neuromuscular blockade (presence of two twitches on TOF monitor) – 2 mg/kg
- For reversal of deep neuromuscular blockade (presence of no TOF twitches but a PTC of 1–2) – 4 mg/kg
- For rescue reversal following rocuronium 1.2 mg/kg – after 3 minutes – 16 mg/kg

Sub-therapeutic doses will result in either incomplete reversal or recurrence of the block. There is no evidence to suggest a difference in reversal time if volatile maintenance has been used, as is the case with neostigmine. The drug may reduce the activity of hormonal contraceptive agents. The effect is thought to be equivalent to taking the pill 12 hours too late.

Mirakhur R. Suggamadex for the reversal of NMB. *Anaesthesia* 2009; **64** (Suppl 1): 45–54

A5

Answer: e.

Anaesthesia for ECT presents a challenge in a remote site. The recommendations from the AAGBI and RCoA are that a consultant should be responsible for the provision of anaesthetic services in this area, but a post-fellowship trainee may undertake the lists as long as they have been trained appropriately and achieved all competencies relating to anaesthesia in this area. They must have access to a fixed telephone line for immediate advice and a consultant must be available to provide assistance if needed. An anaesthetic machine and pipeline oxygen are not mandatory, but there must be a flow-controlled oxygen supply with a reserve supply immediately available. Full monitoring to AAGBI standards is mandatory.

Propofol is anticonvulsant and raises the seizure threshold, but is widely used since the withdrawal of methohexitone (which lowered the seizure threshold). Propofol provides good haemodynamic stability following the surge of sympathetic activity that is produced. Etomidate is sometimes used for resistant cases, but results in less cardiovascular stability. Suxamethonium in a dose of 0.25–1.0 mg/kg is widely used to prevent injury from sudden and forceful muscular contraction produced as a result of the seizure.

Guidance on Provision of Anaesthetic Care in the Non-theatre Environment. RCoA, Revised, 2011.

Anaesthetic Services in Remote Sites. RCoA, London, 2011 (www.rcoa.ac.uk/docs/Remote-sites2011.pdf).

A6

Answer: c.

The increasing demand for the provision of anaesthetic services in the MRI scanner requires the anaesthetist to have a thorough knowledge of the equipment specifications that are required according to the type and strength of the scanner being used.

To avoid ambiguity, the term MRI compatible is no longer used as there have been numerous reports of injuries to patients and staff even with equipment that has been certified as compatible. Two terms are now used as standard to describe the safety of equipment in this environment:

MR conditional refers to an item that has been demonstrated to pose no known hazards in a specified environment with specified conditions of use.

MR safe designated equipment presents no safety hazard to patients or personnel when taken into the MR room providing that instructions concerning its use are correctly followed. There is, however, no guarantee that it will function correctly or not interfere with the image quality produced.

The majority of scanners in the UK generate a field strength of 1.5 tesla (T) but, increasingly, 3-T scanners are being installed and in many cases replacing the older 1.5-T machines. It must not be assumed that equipment conditional at 1.5 T is also conditional at 3 T as this is usually not the case. The main advantage of 3 T systems is improved image quality, but the claims of increased speed and efficiency are debatable. The higher field strength causes more interference with monitoring and the heating effect is much more evident, making them unsuitable for children less than 2 years of age.

Temperature probes can risk conducting heat and causing thermal injury but MR conditional probes are now available.

Association of Anaesthetists of Great Britain and Ireland Guideline 2010. *Safety in Magnetic Resonance Units 2010 – An Update*

A7
Answer: d.

Heparin-induced thrombocytopenia is the development of thrombocytopenia due to the administration of heparin, an anticoagulant. When thrombosis is identified, the condition is called heparin-induced thrombotic thrombocytopenia (HITT).

There are two problems to consider in this question. Firstly, there is the problem of HITT. Secondly, the patient requires renal replacement therapy but has clot formation on the filter membrane reducing its efficiency. As HITT is a prothrombotic condition, it is insufficient to simply stop heparin administration. An alternative anti-coagulant should be prescribed, but the *first-line* strategy would be to administer the fluid pre-filter.

Aspirin is not an option and warfarin should not be administered in the acute setting as there is a risk of skin necrosis. LMWH has less risk of HITT formation than unfractionated heparins but should still be avoided. Alternative anticoagulants include lepirudin and danaparoid.

Danaparoid is an anticoagulant that works by inhibiting activated factor Xa. It is used as a heparinoid substitute in HIT. It can be administered intravenously and may cause throm-bocytopenia. It should be used with caution in asthmatics.

Ahmed I, Majeed A and Powell R. Heparin-induced thrombocytopenia: diagnosis and management update. *Postgrad Med J* 2007; **83**: 575–582

A8
Answer: b.

The interscalene approach to the brachial plexus can be used to provide analgesia for the shoulder, humerus and elbow. It commonly fails to block C8 and T1 and is therefore known as an 'ulnar sparing' block and cannot be used reliably for surgery on the forearm or hand.

The phrenic nerve is blocked in almost all interscalene blocks, so the block should only ever be used on one side at a time. Even one-sided blocks have been shown to have a measurable effect on respiratory mechanics and this should be taken into account when assessing patients and deciding how to proceed.

The stellate ganglion can be blocked in up to 25% of cases. This would result in Horner's syndrome. Five to ten per cent of interscalene blocks result in recurrent laryngeal nerve palsy.

Beecroft CL, Coventry DM. Anaesthesia for shoulder surgery. *Contin Educ Anaesth Crit Care Pain* 2008; **8**(6): 193–198.

A9

Answer: b.

The main cause of the agitation in this ventilated patient is hyponatraemia. Hyponatraemia is a common complication post brain injury and it is essential to find out the underlying cause in order to guide further treatment. The two most important differential diagnoses in a patient with a brain injury are syndrome of inappropriate ADH (SIADH) and cerebral salt-wasting syndrome (CSWS). Both are characterized by low serum sodium and raised urinary sodium and urine osmolality, but there are some important distinctions between the two.

The patient with CSWS produces large volumes of urine which results in plasma volume depletion. They will appear dehydrated and show signs of hypovolaemia (which may explain the tachycardia and hypotension in this case). In SIADH, low volumes of concentrated urine are produced, and patients tend to be euvolaemic.

As a result, the management of the two is extremely different. Whilst SIADH is treated with fluid restriction and demeclocycline 600–1200 mg/day to inhibit the renal response of ADH, CSWS requires restoration of plasma volume and sodium levels. This can be initially done with 0.9% NaCl, although hypertonic saline can be considered. Fludrocortisone 0.1–0.4 mg/day is given in resistant cases for postural hypotension.

Desmopressin is synthetic vasopressin and is used in the treatment of cranial diabetes insipidus and von Willebrand's disease.

Bradshaw K, Smith M. Disorders of sodium balance after brain injury. *Br J Anaesth CEACCP* 2008; **8**: 129–133

A10

Answer: a.

Migraine occurs in 15% of the UK adult population. It is estimated that 190 000 attacks are experienced every day, with three-quarters of those affected reporting disability. Those who suffer migraine attacks typically give an account of recurrent episodic moderate or severe headaches lasting part of a day or up to 3 days and that can be associated with gastrointestinal symptoms. Migraine can also occur with or without an aura with its principal differential diagnosis being tension-type headache.

The evidence for many acute anti-migraine drugs is lacking. For aspirin/metoclopramide in combination, the evidence is better, and for the 'triptans' it is generally good. Recommended analgesic doses for acute migraine are typically greater than standard doses to achieve rapid therapeutic levels against a background of gastric stasis. These drugs should be used without codeine or dihydrocodeine. In fact, narcotics are not recommended for the emergency treatment of migraine as their use can be associated with delayed recovery.

In this question a rapid response is required and sumatriptan subcutaneously is the triptan of choice as only sumatriptan offers this option. However, some specialists favour diclofenac 75 mg intramuscularly, which can be given alone or in combination with an antiemetic. In addition, rehydration with intravenous saline is advisable.

The other options b, d and e are all used in the prophylactic treatment of migraine.

MacGregor EA, Steiner TJ, Davies PTG. *Guidelines for All Health Professionals in the Diagnosis and Management of Migraine*. 3rd edn, 2010. Hull: British Association for the Study of Headache

A11

Answer: e.

Gastrointestinal decontamination is not recommended for routine use in patients subjected to oral poisoning since it may be associated with unpleasant and potentially hazardous side effects. Furthermore, it is very unlikely to be effective beyond 1 hour after poison ingestion.

The most appropriate method for this patient is activated charcoal. Activated charcoal weakly binds most drugs and allows their elimination without absorption. If a dose of 1 g/kg is administered 30 minutes after poisoning, it reduces drug absorption by 90%, reducing to 30% at 1 hour. It should not be administered after 1 hour, nor should it be used in poisoning with the following drugs:

- Iron
- Ethylene glycol
- Lithium
- Methanol
- Acids
- Alkalis
- Corrosive drugs

Repeated doses of activated charcoal at 6-hourly intervals may be of benefit in cases of poisoning with enteric-coated drugs. Ipecacuanha is an emetogenic drug which induces vomiting within 20 minutes of administration. Its use is not recommended by the European Association of Poisons Centres and Clinical Toxicologists.

Whole bowel irrigation with 1.5 to 2 litres/hour of polyethylene glycol is not recommended for routine use in poisoning, though it may be effective when used to treat ingestion of sustained-release preparations.

Gastric lavage has been used to clear the stomach of drug fragments within one hour of drug ingestion, though its use is unsupported by evidence of clinical effectiveness. It may be associated with significant complications such as pulmonary aspiration.

Ward C, Sair M. Oral poisoning: an update. *Contin Educ Anaesth Crit Care Pain* 2010; 6–11.

A12

Answer: a.

The Parkland formula for resuscitation of burns patients is:

- Fluid requirements = TBSA burned(%) x wt (kg) x 4 ml
- (Give half of total requirements in first 8 hours, then give second half over next 16 hours.)
- The fluid administered is Hartmann's solution.

For the purposes of this question you need to estimate the fluid requirements based on total body surface area (TBSA) burned and not just full thickness burn surface area.

Using the rule of 9s the TBSA burned can be calculated:

The Rule of Nines

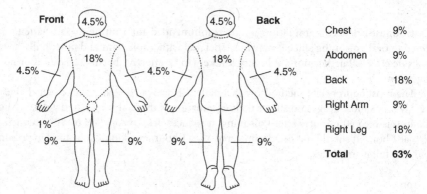

Chest	9%
Abdomen	9%
Back	18%
Right Arm	9%
Right Leg	18%
Total	**63%**

Fig. A12. The rule of nines.

Chest 9%
Abdomen 9%
Back 18%
Right arm 9%
Right leg 18%
TBSA = 63%

Therefore, estimated fluid requirements are:
$63 \times 70 \times 4 = 17\,640$ ml of Hartmann's solution
8820 ml (i.e. half) should be given in the first 8 hours

Bishop S, Maguire S. Anaesthesia and intensive care for major burns. *Contin Educ Anaesth Crit Care Pain* Doi: 10.1093/bjaceaccp/mks001 first published online 23rd February, 2012

A13

Answer: c.

Knowledge of specialized paediatric cardiac surgery is not required for the diploma of the FRCA. However, it does require understanding of the fetal circulation.

HLHS is a rare congenital cardiac lesion characterized by underdevelopment of the left ventricle, outflow tract, mitral valve and aortic valve. The right ventricle receives venous return and ejects into the pulmonary circulation in the normal manner, but the only route for blood to take into the systemic circulation is via the ductus arteriosus (an example of a duct-dependent circulation). The duct can be kept open for the first few days with a prostaglandin infusion, but surgical correction is always required.

Surgical repair occurs in three stages:

1. (Modified) Norwood procedure (neonatal period);
2. Cavopulmonary shunt;
3. Total cavopulmonary connection (usually around 4 years old).

If these patients require critical care or anaesthesia for surgery at a future date, a key aspect of management is to maintain a high circulating volume and central venous pressure as pulmonary blood flow is now dependent on venous pressure and venous return rather than ventricular function.

Barron DJ, Kilby MD, Davies B *et al*. Hypoplastic left heart syndrome. *Lancet* 2009; **374** (15): 551–564

A14

Answer: b.

Fibromyalgia is a chronic pain condition, which is extremely difficult to treat effectively. Treatment in chronic pain clinics has varying success between patients and may be focused more on coping strategies, rather than on analgesia.

A variety of drugs have been trialled with mixed results. TCAs have been shown to be beneficial in some cases. They work by reducing 5-HT reuptake and improve pain as well as sleep in some patients. SSRIs do indeed improve mood. This may have some beneficial effect on the patient's coping skills, but has not been shown to have any benefit in terms of reported pain scores. MAOIs have a wide range of benefits including reduced pain, improved mood and sleeping patterns and reduced daytime fatigue.

Lidocaine infusions are sometimes used but in lower doses than this. Generally, 3–5 mg/ kg is used over 1–2 hours. ECG monitoring and trained assistance are recommended if IV lidocaine is to be used. TENS therapy is a potentially useful form of pain control.

Dedhia JD, Bone ME. Pain and fibromyalgia. *Contin Educ Anaesth Crit Care Pain* 2009; **9** (5): 162–166

A15

Answer: d.

IABP not only improves the function of the left ventricle, but also has a favourable effect on the right ventricle. The pressure gradient between the aorta and the left ventricle increases when the IABP balloon inflates during diastole. This increases the coronary blood flow, hence improving the oxygen delivery to the myocardium. During systole, the balloon deflates, which decreases the afterload of the left ventricle. The coronary blood flow, in patients suffering from severe coronary artery disease depends directly on the diastolic perfusion pressure. Since the IABP increases the diastolic pressure, the coronary blood flow increases in these patients. The increased cardiac output improves the renal blood flow, which may increase up to 25%. The urine output occasionally decreases after initiating the IABP, which may be due to inappropriate placement of the balloon. Haemolysis may decrease the haemoglobin levels and the haematocrit by up to 5%.

Krishna M, Zacharowski K. Principles of intra-aortic balloon pump counterpulsation. *Contin Educ Anaesth Crit Care Pain* 2009; **9**(1): 24–28

A16

Answer: e.

Managing an uncooperative child is a major challenge and requires forethought, particularly if the child has learning difficulties.

The preoperative assessment is a time when reassurance can be offered to both the child and the parents or carers. It is important to adopt a relaxed tone, to use language appropriate for the child's age and to avoid using jargon. In children with mental disorders, establishing a rapport can be difficult. Predictive factors for children who may be distressed at induction include:

- Age between 1 and 3
- Shy, withdrawn behaviour
- Anxious parents
- Previous negative hospital experiences

Management strategies can be psychological and/or pharmacological. Psychological interventions include prehospital visits and play therapy. The presence of a parent at induction is commonplace, though this may be more of benefit to the parent than the child.

The most common sedative used in the UK is midazolam. Following an oral dose of 0.5 mg/kg, a peak effect is seen within 20–30 minutes. It is suitable for both in-patient and day-case surgery. Midazolam can also be given as an intranasal and sublingual preparation.

Ketamine is highly lipid soluble and rapidly absorbed. An oral dose of 5–8 mg/kg will produce a peak effect in 20–25 min. However, this dose can be associated with emergence reactions, particularly after short procedures, and the child will require careful postoperative observation and a quiet environment to recover in.

The physical restraint of children should only be used as an option of last resort and requires the prior agreement of the child's parents. The parents may wish to be involved and minimal force should be used by all involved.

Tan L, Meakin G. Anaesthesia for the uncooperative child. *Cont Educ Anaesth Crit Care Pain* 2010; **10**(2): 48–52

A17

Answer: c.

The pleural space typically contains a small amount of alkaline fluid, pH 7.6, which has a low amount of protein, <1.5 g/l.

Transudates have a protein concentration of <30 g/l and causes include congestive heart failure, nephrotic syndrome, cirrhosis with ascites and peritoneal dialysis.

Exudates have a protein concentration of >30 g/l and causes include malignancy, parapneumonic effusions, PE, connective tissue diseases and subphrenic abscess. Exudative effusions meet at least one of Light's criteria, transudative effusions meet none:

(i) The ratio of pleural fluid protein to serum protein is >0.5;
(ii) The ratio of pleural fluid LDH and serum LDH is >0.6;
(iii) Pleural fluid LDH is more than two-thirds normal upper limit for serum

Paramasivam E, Bodenham A. Pleural fluid collections in critically ill patients. *Contin Educ Anaesth Crit Care Pain* 2007; **7**(1): 10–14

A18

Answer: e.

Patients undergoing amputation are almost certainly going to be left with some persistent phantom phenomena after the procedure. It is thought that changes at the level of both the peripheral and central nervous systems are involved in inducing and maintaining phantom pain. Predictors of phantom pain include lower limb procedures, bilateral amputations, pre-existing pain and adulthood. Though pre-emptive regional anaesthesia might be thought to reduce the risk of persistent phantom pain developing, this has been refuted in the literature. If pre-amputation pain has been existing for some time, a preoperative epidural is unlikely to eradicate the 'memory' of this pain in the central nervous system. The use of tricyclic antidepressants such as amitriptyline and anticonvulsants, namely gabapentin, have the best level of evidence for efficacy in the literature. Ketamine does have some evidence to support its use, though more trials are needed. The benefits of mirror-box therapy and spinal cord stimulation remain unproven. Treatment of phantom limb pain is difficult and combinations of therapies are usually required.

Nikolajsen L. Phantom limb pain, in Stannard CF, Kalso E, Ballantyne J *Evidence-Based Chronic Pain Management*, 1st edn, 2010; Wiley-Blackwell: 237–247

Jackson MA, Simpson KH. Pain after amputation. *Contin Educ Anaesth Crit Care Pain* 2004; 4(1):20–23

A19

Answer: a.

Patients with mild disease may not require specific *Clostridium difficile* antibiotic treatment. If treatment is required, oral metronidazole is recommended (dose: 400–500 mg tds for 10–14 days), as it has been shown to be as effective as oral vancomycin in mild to moderate CDI. For patients with moderate disease, a 10- to 14-day course of oral metronidazole is the recommended treatment (dose: 400–500 mg tds). This is because it is cheaper than oral vancomycin and there is concern that overuse of vancomycin may result in the selection of vancomycin-resistant enterococci. For patients with severe CDI, oral vancomycin is preferable (dose: 125 mg qds for 10–14 days). This is because of relatively high failure rates of metronidazole and a slower clinical response to metronidazole compared with oral vancomycin treatment. No single parameter alone is highly predictive of severe CDI. Current recommendations use any of the following to indicate severe CDI and so to use oral vancomycin in preference to metronidazole:

- WCC >15 × 10^9/l;
- Acutely rising blood creatinine (e.g. >50% increase above baseline)
- Temperature >38.5 °C
- Evidence of severe colitis (abdominal signs, radiology)

In severe CDI cases not responding to oral vancomycin 125 mg qds, high-dose oral vancomycin (up to 500 mg qds) plus intravenous (iv) metronidazole 500 mg tds are recommended.

Department of Health and Health Protection Agency Guidelines. *Clostridium difficile* infection: how to deal with the problem. December 2008

A20

Answer: e.

a. and b. are single low-risk factors for VTE. Fewer than two low-risk factors is not an indication for postnatal thromboprophylaxis. Other low-risk factors include: parity ≥3, smoker, elective C-section, any surgical procedure in the puerperium, gross varicose veins, current systemic infection, immobility, pre-eclampsia, mid-cavity rotational operative delivery, prolonged labour, PPH >1 litre or blood transfusion.

c. and d. are high-risk factors for VTE. Either of these alone would mandate at least 6 weeks postnatal thromboprophylaxis.

e. is an intermediate-risk factor for VTE. Thromboprophylaxis should be continued for at least 7 days postnatally. Other intermediate-risk factors include: asymptomatic thrombophilia, BMI >40, prolonged hospital admission, medical comorbidities, e.g. heart or lung disease, SLE, cancer, IV drug user, two or more low-risk factors.

Green-top Gudeline No. 37a. *Reducing the Risk of Thrombosis and Embolism During Pregnancy and the Puerperium.* RCOG http://www.rcog.org.uk/womens-health/clinical-guidance/reducing-risk-of-thrombosis-greentop37a Accessed 20/02/2012

A21

Answer: c.

In assessing a child with epilepsy it is important to elucidate the cause and nature of the disease in that patient (frequency of seizures, date of last seizure and medication regime). Preoperatively the child may be very anxious and since hyperventilation (hypocarbia) reduces the seizure threshold consideration of benzodiazepine premedication for elective surgery could be made. Clearly intraoperatively normocarbia should also be achieved.

Induction with sevoflurane, nitrous oxide and oxygen in the uncooperative child is not contraindicated; however, the preferable induction technique would be intravenous induction. Sevoflurane may cause epileptiform EEG changes, particularly in higher concentrations or with hypocarbia. Isoflurane is a good choice for maintenance since it suppresses epileptiform EEG activity particularly at >1 MAC and causes isoelectric EEG at >2 MAC.

Hepatic enzyme induction secondary to medication leads to resistance to non-depolarizing neuromuscular blockers, and their dose and frequency may need to be increased. Large doses or prolonged infusions of atracurium should be avoided since the metabolite, laudanosine, has epileptogenic potential.

There have been concerns that regional blockade may reduce the seizure threshold or confuse the clinical picture by risking convulsions from toxicity. They are not contraindicated, however. Alfentanil and the metabolites of pethidine are epileptogenic and should be avoided.

Intraoperatively, the anaesthetist should be vigilant to the possibility of masked or non-convulsive seizure activity. Signs may be ambiguous, such as sudden unexplained increases in end-tidal carbon dioxide, tachycardia, hypertension, increased muscle tone, pupil dilatation and increased oxygen consumption. Treatment involves administering 100% oxygen, deepening anaesthesia (+/- administration of an anticonvulsant such as propofol, thiopentone or benzodiazepine) and correcting precipitant factors (hypoxia, hypocarbia or hypoglycaemia).

Barakat, A, Mallory, S. Anaesthesia and childhood epilepsy. *Contin Educ Anaesth Crit Care Pain* 2011; 11(3): 93–98

A22

Answer: e.

The peril of chronic pain management is to fail to recognize an organic cause for pain, such as a malignancy or cauda equina syndrome. 'Red flags' are elements of a patient history or examination that are suggestive of a serious underlying pathology. The red flags in the given scenario are his age, his sensory disturbance and his use of mesalazine, a mild immunosuppressant.

Red flag conditions and the symptoms associated with them are given below:

Cauda equina syndrome	Saddle anaesthesia Sphincter disturbance Progressive motor/sensory disturbance
Tumour/infection	Presentation <20 or >55 years Rest pain/night pain/thoracic pain Systemically unwell/fever Unexplained weight loss Immunosuppression, HIV, iv drug use
Fracture	Trauma Osteoporosis

Jackson MA, Simpson KH. Chronic back pain. *Contin Educ Anaesth Crit Care Pain* 2006; 6(4): 152–155

A23

Answer: e.

In obese patients, the volume of the central compartment is unchanged, but the volume of distribution of the highly fat-soluble drugs such as barbiturates increases greatly. For such drugs, the induction dose should be based on ideal body weight (IBW), as their peak plasma concentration is the same as when the dose is adjusted according to the patient's cardiac output.

Propofol, despite being a highly fat-soluble drug is not dosed according to the IBW but as per total body weight (TBW), as it has a very high clearance. At a steady state, its volume of distribution and clearance are relative to TBW. The same is true when using propofol infusions for TIVA.

Neuromuscular blocking drugs are water soluble and have a negligible change in the volume of distribution. Dosing by lean body weight (LBW) is more accurate (LBW = IBW + 20%). Suxamethonium doses, when used for rapid sequence induction should be calculated according to the TBW as it ensures good conditions for intubation.

Local anaesthetics should be calculated as per the IBW due to the risk of toxicity at higher doses. When used neuraxially, the dose should be decreased by 25%. This is because the volume of the epidural space in the obese is reduced due to presence of excess fat and engorged veins. The appropriate dosing scale for most anaesthetic drugs including opioids in the obese is usually LBW.

Lotia S, Bellamy MC. Anaesthesia and morbid obesity. *Contin Educ Anaesth Crit Care Pain* 2008; **8**(5): 151–156

Ingrade J, Lemmens HJM. Dose adjustment of anaesthetics in the morbidly obese. *Br J Anaesth* 2010; **105**(Suppl 1): i16–i23

A24

Answer: c.

Red cell alloimmunization is most likely to occur in the third trimester. Accordingly, no pretransfusion blood sample should be more than 7 days old and ideally, should be fresh. Kell-negative blood should be used for transfusion in women of child-bearing age, unless that woman is already Kell-positive. FFP or cryoprecipitate may contain small amounts of red cell stroma, but sensitization is most unlikely as stroma is less immunogenic than intact red cells, therefore anti-D prophylaxis is not required following Rh-positive FFP or cryoprecipitate transfusion. The platelet count should not be allowed to fall below 50×10^9/l in the acutely bleeding patient; however, a transfusion trigger of 75×10^9/l is recommended to provide a safety margin.

Rege K, Bamber J, Slack MC. *et al.* 2008. *Blood Transfusion in Obstetrics.* London: Royal College of Obstetricians and Gynaecologists

British Committee for Standards in Haematology Blood Transfusion Task Force. Guidelines for the use of FFP, cryoprecipitate and cryosupernatant. *Br J Haematol* 2004; **126**: 11–28.

A25

Answer: e.

CRT (biventricular pacing) may have a role to play in patients with LBBB. Restrictive cardiomyopathy does not usually require manipulation of the coordinated electrical activity of the heart. In some situations it may become appropriate, but there is simply not enough information in option d. to justify it as single best answer. CRT is of no specific benefit in the patient with valvular heart disease or supraventricular dysrhythmias. An automated internal cardiac defibrillator (AICD) would be more appropriate in the patient with recurrent VT.

Zareba W, Klein H, Cygankiewicz I. *et al.* Effectiveness of cardiac resynchronization therapy by QRS morphology in the multicenter automatic defibrillator implantation trial – cardiac resynchronization therapy (MADIT-CRT). *Circulation* 2011; **123**(10): 1061–1072

A26

Answer: b.

The simple definition of postoperative cognitive dysfunction (POCD) would be a long-term, possibly permanent, disabling deterioration in cognitive function following surgery. The risk of prolonged POCD is approximately 10% following major surgery in patients over 60 years of age and the incidence may be as high as one in three in patients over 80 years of age. The aetiology of POCD is unclear. Mechanisms such as perioperative hypoxaemia and ischaemia have been suggested but, surprisingly, this is not supported by evidence. Also, regional anaesthesia (in the place of general anaesthesia) probably reduces early POCD but not prolonged POCD. Increased inflammatory activity may play a role in early POCD – elevated C-reactive protein is associated with cognitive dysfunction in hip fracture patients.

Predisposing factors for POCD:

Early POCD	Prolonged POCD
Increasing age	Increasing age only
GA rather than RA	
Duration of anaesthesia	
Lower level of education	
Reoperation	
Postoperative infection	

An awareness of the issue of POCD is essential, particularly when contemplating major surgery in the elderly and the issue should be discussed with patients and their families.

Fines DP, Severn AM. Anaesthesia and cognitive disturbance in the elderly. *Contin Educ Anaesth Crit Care Pain* 2006; **6** (1): 37–40

Deiner S, Silverstein JH. Postoperative delirium and cognitive dysfunction. *Br J Anaesth* 2009; **103** (Suppl 1): i41–i46

A27

Answer: d.

Polydipsia in diabetics results from fluid loss due to the osmotic diuretic effect of raised glucose. This is also the mechanism by which DKA produces dehydration and leads to acidosis. As treatment is introduced, plasma glucose falls below the renal threshold. Polyuria resolves as glucose no longer exerts an osmotic effect from within the renal tubules. As polyuria decreases and fluids are replaced, thirst, and therefore polydipsia, also resolve.

Patients may have sympathetic or parasympathetic autonomic neuropathy, or both. In those with parasympathetic neuropathy, the normal sinus arrhythmia associated with inspiration is reduced.

Regional blocks are useful in diabetic patients as they reduce the stress response and can aid postoperative glucose control. There is debate whether adrenaline should be used, as blood supply may already be compromised to the periphery.

Pain is associated with a stress response. In diabetic patients the stress response can increase insulin requirements. This is one reason for placing patients on a 'sliding scale' infusion if they are undergoing major surgery.

Occult infections are present in over 15% of diabetic patients.

Flynn MD, O'Brien IA, Corrall RJ. The prevalence of autonomic and peripheral neuropathy in insulin-treated diabetic subjects. *Diabet Med* 1995; **12**: 310–313

Williams BA, Murinson BB. Diabetes mellitus and subclinical neuropathy: a call for new paths in peripheral nerve block research. *Anesthesiology* 2008; **109**: 361–362

A28

Answer: b.

Patients with bronchopleural fistulas have a persistent leak, which interferes with re-expansion of the lung in spite of a chest drain. The mainstay of treatment in these patients is maintaining oxygenation and ventilation and decreasing the air leak through the fistula. Most fistulae heal spontaneously with time, over a few days. The ventilation strategy includes using low tidal volumes and respiratory rate along with low inspiratory pressures, inspiratory times and low PEEP. In these patients, one should accept permissive hypercapnia and low oxygen saturations.

Paramasivam E, Bodenham A. Air leaks, pneumothorax and chest drains. *Contin Educ Anaesth Crit Care Pain* 2008; 8(6): 204–209

A29

Answer: c.

The total incidence including perioperative cases is between one and two per thousand population per year. Pulmonary embolism is under-diagnosed in the perioperative period.

The value of the D-dimer test is in exclusion rather than confirmation of the diagnosis. A low D-dimer makes thromboembolism an unlikely diagnosis. High D-dimers can be caused by a range of pathologies (such as surgery itself) and are not necessarily proof of thromboembolism. CTPA is now the investigation of choice in suspected PTE. Most departments will be able to organize them fairly rapidly, but anti-coagulation should not be delayed as the condition has a mortality of around 30%, with around 10% dying acutely within the first hour after the embolism. Patients who are too unstable to have a CTPA should have bedside echocardiography and, if PTE or right heart failure is detected, they should be considered for thrombolysis on this basis. Haemodynamic instability is uncommon except in massive PTE, which accounts for around 5% of the total number of cases.

Patients with large but not total occlusion (around 25% of cases) may be haemodynamically stable, but will often show signs such as right heart strain on echocardiograms. Vena cava filters have been shown in some studies to increase VTE. They are used in cases where interim prophylaxis is required and anticoagulant therapy would be hazardous.

ESC Task Force for the Diagnosis and Management of Acute Pulmonary Embolism Guidelines on the diagnosis and management of acute pulmonary embolism. *Eur Heart J* 2008; **29**: 2276–2315

Van Beek EJR, Elliot CA, Kiely DG. Diagnosis and initial treatment of patients with suspected pulmonary thromboembolism. *Contin Educ Anaesth Crit Care Pain* 2009; **9** (4): 119–124

A30

Answer: a.

Saline-soaked gauze will *reduce*, but not eliminate the risk of fire. Smoke evacuation is to reduce the risk of combustion, not to protect the surgeon. Maintaining a low F_iO_2 to reduce the risk of combustion is more important than using methylene blue to signal cuff rupture. Double cuff laser tubes are also available.

Schramm VL Jr, Mattox DE, Stool SE. Acute management of laser-ignited intratracheal explosion. *Laryngoscope* 1981; **91**(9,1): 1417–1426

Paper B – Questions

B1

A 45-year-old male returns from theatre after quadruple bypass surgery. He has a pulmonary artery catheter *in situ* and develops a sustained ventricular tachycardia as you attempt to float the catheter.

The most appropriate step in management would be:
a. Administration of intravenous amiodarone
b. Electrical cardioversion
c. Removal of the catheter tip from the right ventricle
d. Correction of electrolytes
e. Administration of intravenous lidocaine

B2

A 38-year-old alcoholic male is admitted with severe upper abdominal pain of 24 hours' duration. Infected peri-pancreatic necrosis is confirmed on a computed tomography scan.

The most appropriate initial management is:
a. Immediate laparotomy and pancreatic resection
b. Percutaneous drainage of necrotic tissue
c. Endoscopic retrograde cholangiopancreatography (ERCP)
d. Conservative treatment with broad spectrum antibacterials
e. Minimally invasive retroperitoneal approach to pancreatic resection

B3

A 55-year-old female with previous mitral valve replacement (mechanical valve) for rheumatic heart disease presents with a 3-week history of increasing lethargy and intermittent febrile episodes. Blood cultures have grown *Staphylococcus aureus* and she has been commenced on flucloxacillin. A transthoracic echocardiogram performed on admission demonstrated a normal-looking mitral valve prosthesis. Following a period of initial improvement, she becomes more unwell, developing increasing dyspnoea, tachycardia (heart rate 130 and irregular) and embolic phenomena such as peripheral vasculitic lesions.

What is the next best step?
a. Consent for mitral valve repair

Practice Single Best Answer Questions for the Final FRCA, ed. Hozefa Ebrahim, Khalid Hasan, Mark Tindall, Michael Clarke and Natish Bindal. Published by Cambridge University Press. © Cambridge University Press 2013.

b. Consent for mitral valve replacement
c. Repeat blood cultures to detect the emergence of multi-resistant organisms
d. Arrange for a repeat transthoracic echocardiogram
e. Arrange for a transoesphageal echocardiogram

B4

A 78-year-old female has undergone an aortic valve replacement 6 hours previously. She is hypotensive with increasing vasopressor requirements and her central venous pressures are elevated. She develops a severe bradycardia and you are unable to feel a carotid pulse. There is no response to 3 mg of atropine administered via a central line or to epicardial pacing.

The next most appropriate step would be:
a. Increase epicardial pacing output
b. Administration of isoprenaline
c. Administration of fluid challenge
d. Emergency resternotomy
e. Correction of electrolytes

B5

You are called to the emergency department to see a 45-year-old male who has been found in his garage with his car engine running. His face is a cherry-red colour in appearance, he has a GCS of 12 and the pulse oximeter reads 100% whilst breathing room air.

Your initial priority would be to:
a. Intubate and ventilate the patient
b. Make arrangements for transfer to a facility capable of providing hyperbaric oxygen therapy
c. Deliver high flow (15 litres/minute) oxygen via a non-rebreathe mask
d. Check blood glucose level
e. Administer intravenous steroids to reduce airway oedema

B6

You are called to the emergency department to see a 30-year-old male who has a history of intravenous drug use. He has been found semiconscious on the floor at home. His friend states that he is unsure how long he had been lying on the floor. His creatinine kinase result is 5000 units/l. The arterial blood gas shows pH 7.28, pO_2 13.5 kPa, pCO_2 3.3 kPa and K^+ 5.5 mmol/l.

The initial most appropriate management step would be to:
a. Administer 50 ml 50% glucose with 10 iu insulin
b. Administer 100 mmol of 8.4% sodium bicarbonate
c. Administer 100 mg iv furosemide
d. Increase fluid administration to maintain a urine output of >100 ml/hour
e. Start renal replacement therapy

B7

A previously well 9-year-old boy presents to the emergency department with diabetic ketoacidosis. His initial pH was 7.1 with a pCO_2 <2 kPa and lactate 1. He is initially treated with insulin and fluid replacement. He receives 40 ml/kg of 0.9% saline over 3 hours. You are called to review because he has become increasingly drowsy.

What is the most likely cause of his deterioration?
a. Hypoglycaemia
b. Cerebral oedema
c. Hypernatraemia
d. Hypokalaemia
e. Exhaustion

B8

While on-call for the labour ward, you attend a cardiac arrest of a 33-year-old woman. Thirty minutes earlier, you inserted an epidural for labour analgesia. On arrival, CPR is in progress, it appears that the epidural-giving set has been mistakenly connected to the patient's peripheral cannula.

Which of the following would be considered correct in this patient's management?
a. 2% lipid emulsion, given as an initial bolus of 1.5 ml/kg, with a maximum of four repeat boluses
b. 2% lipid emulsion, given as an initial bolus of 1.5 ml/kg over 1 minute, with repeat doses not exceeding 15 ml/kg per hour
c. 2% lipid emulsion, given as an initial bolus of 1.5 ml/kg over 1 minute, followed by an infusion at 30 ml/kg per hour
d. 20% lipid emulsion, given as an initial bolus of 1.5 ml/kg over 1 minute, followed by an infusion at 15 ml/kg per hour
e. 20% lipid emulsion, given as an initial bolus of 1.5 ml over 1 minute, with a maximum of three further repeat boluses

B9

All anaesthetic drugs are associated with cardiovascular changes. Optimizing patient outcomes requires knowledge of the effects of particular agents, how to offset them and when they might be advantageous.

Regarding anaesthetic agents, which statement is most correct?
a. At three times the MAC, all anaesthetic vapours cause coronary steal
b. Anaesthetic preconditioning reduces postoperative myocardial infarction
c. All anaesthetic vapours cause a degree of myocardial damage
d. All anaesthetic vapours are cardioprotective
e. All opioids are cardioprotective

B10

You are assessing a 39-year-old male in your chronic pain management clinic. He gives you a 6-month history of pain in his lower back. There is no history of trauma and he is otherwise well. Your examination is unremarkable. He takes regular paracetamol and ibuprofen, which slightly ease the pain.

After discussing analgesic options, what would be the next step in your management of this patient?
a. Offer a course of physical therapy

27

b. Offer transcutaneous electrical nerve stimulation (TENS)
c. Prescribe gabapentin
d. Request a lumbar spine MRI
e. Request a lumbar spine X-ray

B11

With regard to intraoperative cell salvage (ICS), which of the following statements is true?
a. Malignant disease is an absolute contraindication to the use of ICS
b. NICE have not approved the use of ICS during obstetric haemorrhage
c. It is not safe to aspirate iodine into the ICS system
d. It is safe to aspirate all antibiotics into the ICS system
e. Jehovah's Witnesses will not accept transfusion with ICS blood

B12

Acromegaly is an important anaesthetic consideration.

Which of the following statements regarding acromegaly is most accurate?
a. It is caused by excessive growth hormone secretion before fusion of the epiphysial plates at puberty
b. It is associated with hypoglycaemia due to the effects of growth hormone on the beta cells of the pancreas
c. Upper airway obstruction is unusual because the structures of the oropharynx are larger than normal
d. Supplemental thyroxine may be required because TSH release is reduced.
e. Treatment is by hypophysectomy but care must be taken to avoid giving steroids intraoperatively as the adrenals are hypertrophied in these individuals.

B13

Cardioplegia solutions are primarily used to arrest myocardial contraction and facilitate cardiac surgery. They have a number of other important properties, and knowledge of the type of cardioplegia to be used along with the delivery method can influence anaesthetic delivery.

Which of the following is the most accurate statement?
a. Retrograde cardioplegia delivery requires a competent aortic valve
b. Cardioplegia should be slightly hypo-osmolar
c. Anterograde cardioplegia delivery produces more rapid cardiac arrest than retrograde
d. Cold cardioplegia reduces reperfusion injury
e. Cardioplegia requires around 12 mmol/l of potassium

B14

During an emergency repair of an abdominal aortic aneurysm, your strategy to reduce the risk of postoperative renal impairment involves:
a. Maintaining an adequate extracellular fluid volume and perfusion pressure
b. A dose of 40 mg of furosemide just before the aortic clamp goes on
c. A dose of mannitol of 0.25 mg/kg after induction
d. Dopamine at 3 µg/kg/min
e. Maintaining a central venous pressure of 4–7 mmHg

B15

You are asked to see a lady in the recovery area. She has a history of hyperthyroidism and has just undergone a knee arthroscopy under general anaesthesia. She had to undergo a rapid sequence induction for gastro-oesophageal reflux disease. She is tachycardic, hypertensive, has a temperature of 40 °C and is agitated. Her muscle tone is flaccid and she is also vomiting. The mainstay of your management plan is:
a. Administration of analgesia and an antiemetic, as she may be in pain
b. Administration of 2–3 mg/kg of dantrolene sodium IV, as this may be malignant hyperthermia
c. Re-intubation and sedation until the cause of the problem can be ascertained
d. Propranolol in 1-mg increments, hydrocortisone and propylthiouracil, as this may be a thyroid storm
d. Administration of 50 µg/kg of neostigmine, as she may be inadequately reversed

B16

You are asked to review a child who has undergone a tonsillectomy two hours ago.

Which of the following statements is most accurate, with regards to a post-tonsillectomy bleed?
a. Primary haemorrhage is often due to NSAID use
b. Secondary haemorrhage is more likely to result in hypovolaemic shock than primary haemorrhage
c. If the patient was intubated without difficulty at their first anaesthetic it is unlikely that the airway will present difficulty now
d. Gas induction with sevoflurane is reasonable despite the presence of blood in the stomach
e. Rapid sequence induction is mandatory because the patient cannot be adequately starved

B17

You are asked to assess a patient in the obstetric clinic who has von Willebrand's disease. She is keen to have an epidural for labour if required. There are several types of this disease.

Which type commonly gets *better* during pregnancy?
a. Type 1
b. Type 2A
c. Type 2B
d. Type 2M
e. Type 3

B18

The anhepatic phase of liver transplantation is associated with many physiological derangements.

Which of the following best describes these derangements and the subsequent management?
a. Hypocalcaemia with myocardial depression may develop secondary to the citrate load from blood products and the inability to metabolize it. This can be treated with calcium administration

b. A low cardiac output, which should be corrected with aggressive fluid management
c. A progressive metabolic alkalaemia, treated with acetozolamide
d. Fibrinolysis, which is prevented by administration of antifibrinolytic drugs
e. The absence of production of clotting factors, which necessitates immediate administration of FFP

B19

A 23-year-old, female, ex-intravenous drug user attends the pain clinic with a 3-month history of lower back pain, which does not radiate down the lower limbs. There is no history of trauma, nor are there any features of cauda equina syndrome.

What should be done next?
a. Advise physiotherapy
b. Offer a TENS machine
c. Start on amitriptyline 10 mg po nocte
d. Arrange an MRI scan of the lumbar spine
e. Refer for pain management programme

B20

An unwell 17-year-old girl with a Fontan circulation is listed for an appendicectomy for suspected perforated appendicitis.

Which of the following is is contraindicated in the management of this patient?
a. Giving 10 ml/kg fluid bolus pre-operatively
b. Maintaining a heart rate of less than 60 bpm
c. Antibiotics prophylaxis
d. Intubation and mechanical ventilation during surgery
e. Rapid sequence induction

B21

The diagnostic criteria of acute lung injury (ALI) and acute respiratory distress syndrome (ARDS) differ when describing:
a. The rate of onset
b. The chest X-ray appearance
c. The pulmonary artery wedge pressure
d. The P_aO_2/F_iO_2 ratio
e. The presence of fever

B22

Delirium is a frequent complication of intensive care that prolongs ICU and hospital stay. It can be caused by, or worsened by, drugs, pathology or situational factors.

Which statement is most accurate?
a. Delirium is defined as a change in consciousness developing over a short time period
b. In patients who cannot take haloperidol, benzodiazepines are the first line treatment of delirium
c. Patients with delirium related to acute illness are at high risk of developing a chronic cognitive deficit

d. Patients who smoke 20 or more cigarettes per day have a reduced risk of delirium related to sedation in the ICU

e. Delirium and schizophrenia share diagnostic features and are treated in the same way, but occur over different time scales

B23

Intrathecal opioids have proven extremely useful in both prolonging the duration of spinal anaesthesia and in reducing total doses of local anaesthetics.

Which of the following is most accurate?

a. Intrathecal morphine is associated with respiratory depression after discharge from recovery

b. Intrathecal phenylpiperidine derivatives are not associated with pruritus

c. Morphine has a high volume of distribution within the CSF and is therefore more dilute with a lower side effect profile than more lipophilic opioids.

d. Pethidine is hypobaric and can be used as a sole agent as long as the patient is placed in the Trendelenburg position

e. 5–10 micrograms of fentanyl are required to provide reliable anaesthesia for Caesarean section

B24

A 9-year-old patient is fitting. The nurse says the patient is recovering from a chest infection, but is also known to have epilepsy. The drug chart at the end of the bed shows that the patient is on phenytoin and levetirecetam. The nurse applies high-flow oxygen. There is no iv access *in situ*.

Which of the following is the most appropriate course of action (assuming seizure activity continues)?

a. Spend up to 5 minutes gaining iv/io access, give iv/io lorazepam 0.1 mg/kg, give iv phenytoin 20 mg/kg

b. Spend up to 5 minutes gaining iv/io access, give iv lorazepam 0.1 mg/kg, give iv phenobarbitone 20 mg/kg

c. Give rectal diazepam 0.5 mg/kg, gain iv/io access, give iv lorazepam 0.1 mg/kg, give iv phenytoin 20 mg/kg

d. Give rectal diazepam 0.5 mg/kg, gain iv/io access, give iv lorazepam 0.1 mg/kg, give iv phenytoin 20 mg/kg

e. Give buccal midazolam, 0.5 mg/kg, gain iv/io access, give iv lorazepam 0.1 mg/kg, give iv phenytoin 20 mg/kg

B25

A 19-year-old male patient with known sickle cell disease presents for urgent humeral nailing after falling off his bicycle. Full blood count reveals an Hb of 6.9 g/dl. The orthopaedic team decides to resuscitate him by transfusing with two units of packed red blood cells prior to surgery. The patient becomes tachycardic, and complains of difficulty breathing, but denies chest pain.

The most likely cause is:

a. Sickle chest syndrome

b. Transfusion-related acute lung injury (TRALI)
c. Acute haemolytic transfusion reaction
d. Acute pulmonary oedema following transfusion-associated circulatory overload (TACO)
e. Fat embolism syndrome

B26

You are managing a 30-year-old male admitted to ICU 2 hours ago due to polytrauma following a road traffic collision. He had a prolonged extraction time and his CK is 20 000 u/l. His urine output has been <30 ml/h for the last 2 hours.

Your first action would be:
a. Give frusemide 80 mg iv
b. Resuscitation with 0.9% saline and check his plasma potassium
c. Institute alkalinization of the urine by infusion of 1.26% sodium bicarbonate
d. Insert a vascath and commence haemodiafiltration
e. Give mannitol

B27

A non-diabetic patient attends pre-assessment clinic after being listed for spinal surgery. He informs the nurse that he has been diagnosed with neuropathic pain in his left leg for which he currently takes co-codamol; two tablets four times a day. His symptoms are not controlled and you are phoned for advice.

Which of the following drugs is the most appropriate first-line treatment?
a. Tramadol
b. Amitriptyline
c. Oxycodone
d. Lidocaine patches
e. Duloxetine

B28

A previously fit and well 50-year-old male underwent a decompressive craniectomy for an acute subdural haematoma following a traumatic head injury 24 hours ago. He is now on the neurosurgical intensive care unit and remains intubated and ventilated. You have been asked to review his urine output, which is recorded as 800 ml over the last 2 hours, despite appropriate intravenous fluid administration. You suspect neurogenic diabetes insipidus.

Which of the following features would support your diagnosis?
a. Urine specific gravity >1.005
b. Serum Na^+ <135 mmol/l
c. Urine osmolality <350 mmol/kg
d. Serum osmolality <295 mmol/kg
e. Serum creatinine 200 mmol/l

B29

Transversus abdominis plane (TAP) blocks have recently gained popularity for the provision of analgesia after a range of surgical procedures. A 70-kg patient is listed for a total abdominal hysterectomy, for whom a TAP block is planned.

Which of the following is most accurate?
a. The aim of a TAP block is to place local anaesthetic between the peritoneum and the transversus abdominis muscle
b. 40 ml of local anaesthetic is required for each side
c. A spinal needle is used to perform the block
d. The triangle of Petit is bounded inferiorly by the iliac crest
e. Analgesia can be achieved from T6 to L1 with a single injection

B30

A 24-year-old known asthmatic presents to the emergency department with an acute asthma attack. She has received two boluses of 5 mg of salbutamol via a nebulizer, nebulized ipratropium bromide and hydrocortisone. Despite these measures, she has failed to improve. You are called to assist in her management. Your examination reveals a respiratory rate of $35\,\text{min}^{-1}$, heart rate of $100\,\text{min}^{-1}$, inability to complete one sentence and diffuse wheeze.

Which of the following is the most appropriate management?
a. Continuous nebulized salbutamol
b. Nebulized adrenaline
c. Intravenous salbutamol
d. Increased bolus dose nebulized salbutamol (10 mg)
E. Combined nebulized and intravenous salbutamol.

Paper B – Answers

B1

Answer: c.

The flow-directed balloon-tipped pulmonary artery catheter (PAC) (also known as the Swan–Ganz or right heart catheter) has been in clinical use for more than 30 years.

The development of brief, transient ventricular ectopics is common during passage of the catheter through the right ventricle (RV) and usually subsides once the catheter reaches the pulmonary artery (PA). Sustained ventricular dysrhythmias can be prevented by assuring that the balloon is fully inflated during passage of the catheter from the right atrium (RA) to the PA and by minimizing the insertion time.

Treatment of sustained ventricular tachycardia includes prompt removal of the catheter from the RV (either out to the PA or back to the RA) and administration of lidocaine, if the dysrhythmia persists. The development of ventricular fibrillation requires defibrillation.

Bersten A, Soni N. *Oh's Intensive Care Manual*. 6th ed. Elsevier Limited, 2009

B2

Answer: d.

A randomized controlled trial by Mier *et al.* comparing early vs. delayed surgical intervention in peri-pancreatic necrosis showed better outcomes with a delayed approach. The selection of the most appropriate method for source control must weigh up the risks and benefits of the proposed procedure. Source control interventions, such as laparotomy, can themselves result in further complications such as organ damage, fistula formation and haemorrhage.

Percutaneous drainage of necrotic pancreatic tissue has been attempted, but is not reliably effective due to the tendency for drains to become blocked.

There is some evidence that a minimally invasive retroperitoneal surgical approach may offer advantages in terms of improved outcome, compared with open laparotomy.

ERCP would not be effective unless the cause was due to gallstones.

Mier J, Leon EL, Castillo A, *et al.* Early versus late necrosectomy in severe necrotizing pancreatitis. *Am J Surg* 1997; **173**:71–75

Practice Single Best Answer Questions for the Final FRCA, ed. Hozefa Ebrahim, Khalid Hasan, Mark Tindall, Michael Clarke and Natish Bindal. Published by Cambridge University Press. © Cambridge University Press 2013.

Dellinger RP, Levy MM, Carlet JM, *et al.* Surviving sepsis campaign: International guidelines for management of severe sepsis and septic shock. *Crit Care Med* 2008; **36**: 296–327

B3

Answer: e.

The clinical picture is highly suggestive of prosthetic valve SBE. The best investigation to confirm the diagnosis is TOE whose sensitivity is far greater than TTE, particularly with the mitral valve. Although she is likely to require an emergent MVR, other valvular lesions and the presence of any intracardiac shunts should be sought. In the likely event of needing urgent surgery, the finessing of antimicrobial therapy is less pressing.

Baddour LM, Wilson WR, Bayer AS, *et al.* Infective endocarditis: diagnosis, antimicrobial therapy, and management of complications: a statement for healthcare professionals from the Committee on Rheumatic Fever, Endocarditis, and Kawasaki Disease, Council on Cardiovascular Disease in the Young. *Circulation* 2005; **111**(23): e394–434.

B4

Answer: d.

Cardiac surgical patients who present with a non-VF/VT rhythm are most likely to have a tamponade, tension pneumothorax or severe hypovolaemia. Prompt treatment is associated with an excellent outcome in comparison with non-cardiac surgical patients. Once atropine and pacemaker intervention are found to be ineffective, emergency resternotomy should be undertaken.

Cardiac tamponade requires resternotomy and is the commonest cause of non-VF/VT arrest after cardiac surgery. Tension pneumothorax may be diagnosed by assessment of breathing during basic life support, but it will be promptly relieved during emergency resternotomy if undetected clinically. Hypovolaemia, which causes the patient to suffer a cardiac arrest, will invariably need resternotomy for control of bleeding.

Dunning J, Versteegh M, Fabbri A, *et al.* Guideline for resuscitation of patients who arrest after cardiac surgery. *The Cardiac Surgery Advanced Life Support Course. Course Manual*, 2010

B5

Answer: c.

The diagnosis of carbon monoxide (CO) poisoning is made by a history of exposure and direct measurement of carboxyhaemoglobin (COHb) in the blood. CO and O_2 both bind to the α-chain of the haemoglobin molecule, but CO has 250 times the affinity for the ferrous iron complex compared with O_2. Competitive dissociation of CO from haem binding sites and provision of dissolved oxygen to the tissues is believed to combine to reduce the sequelae of CO poisoning. The half-life of COHb is as follows:

- In air (21% O_2)   240 minutes
- 100% O_2 (1 atmosphere) 40 minutes
- 100 O_2 (3 atmospheres) 23 minutes

It can be seen from these figures that simply administering high flow (100% O_2) will increase the speed of CO removal significantly. Hyperbaric oxygen therapy, which can provide nearly all the body's oxygen needs through dissolved oxygen, is often impractical and not necessary in such cases. Since the patient's GCS is 12, there is no immediate need to intubate him, although he should be nursed in a high dependency area with a low threshold for intubation if signs of airway compromise develop. A bronchoscopy may be performed at a later stage if the patient needs intubation. There are no direct data supporting steroid use in smoke inhalation and due to the increased risk of infection and delayed wound healing, prolonged use of steroids is discouraged.

Hawkins M, Harrison J, Charters P. Severe carbon monoxide poisoning: outcome after hyperbaric oxygen therapy. *Br J Anaesth* 2000; **84**(5): 584–586

B6

Answer: d.

Vigorous hydration with isotonic crystalloid is the cornerstone of therapy for rhabdomyolysis. Support of the intravascular volume increases the glomerular filtration rate and oxygen delivery as well as diluting myoglobin and other renal tubular toxins. Injured myocytes can sequester large volumes of extracellular fluid and so crystalloid requirements may be surprisingly high.

Mannitol can be given to maintain a diuresis once intravascular fluid volume is adequate. Furosemide has been used in this way to maintain a diuresis, but it can acidify the urine. Urinary alkalinization with sodium bicarbonate helps to increase the solubility of myoglobin. With ongoing renal failure, renal support may be necessary in the form of renal replacement therapy.

Better OS, Stein JH. Early management of shock and prophylaxis of acute renal failure in traumatic rhabdomyolysis. *N Engl J Med* 1990; **322**(12):825–829

B7

Answer: b.

Management of paediatric diabetic ketoacidosis (DKA) is broadly similar to that in adults, namely administration of insulin, fluids and replacement of electrolytes. The key differences are that children often present with greater severity and they have a greater predilection to develop cerebral oedema.

Cerebral oedema occurs in up to 1% of all paediatric DKA episodes and accounts for 60%–90% of all DKA deaths. Risk factors include: young age, newly diagnosed diabetes, raised serum urea, initial pH<7.1, extreme hypocapnia (pCO_2<2 kPA) and >40 ml/kg total fluid given in the first 4 hours.

Fluid therapy involves fluid resuscitation to replace inadequate intravascular volume and replacing the fluid deficit secondary to dehydration. Shock with haemodynamic compromise is uncommon in DKA and judicious use of fluid is advised. It is rare to require more than 20 ml/kg fluid in the first 1–2 hours. Rehydration should occur slowly over a minimum of 48 hours and hypotonic solutions should be avoided due to the risk of cerebral oedema.

If cerebral oedema is suspected, then treatment should start immediately with either hypertonic saline 3% or mannitol and an urgent head CT should be arranged.

Steel S, Tibby S. Paediatric diabetic ketoacidosis. *Contin Educ Anaesth Crit Care Pain* 2009; **9**(6): 194–199

B8

Answer: d.

Guidelines for the management of severe local anaesthetic toxicity have been published by the AAGBI. See Figure B8 overleaf.

B9

Answer: d.

All anaesthetic vapours are beneficial and cardioprotective at even relatively low concentrations with this effect also including ischaemic tissues. The maximal benefit is thought to occur at around 1.5–2 MAC.

Anaestheic preconditioning results in lower inotrope requirements, better cardiac indices and shorter hospital stays, but has no effect on postoperative MI. Morphine is known to be cardioprotective, but the effect is mediated by the delta opioid receptor and is not common to all opioids.

Ketamine is unique among anaesthetic agents in that it produces a sympathomimetic response causing tachycardia and increased blood pressure. This response is poorly understood and is thought to be centrally mediated. In cases of autonomic dysfunction, ketamine has a direct myocardial depressant effect, but in normal individuals the depressant effect is more than outweighed by the central response.

Nitrous oxide has a direct myocardial depressant effect, but causes an increase in sympathetic outflow which balances this. It causes relatively little change in cardiac output or blood pressure, but it does increase pulmonary vascular resistance, which can lead to right ventricular failure in patients already suffering from pulmonary hypertension.

Modern opioid classification

The history of opiods is long and interesting and has led to a complex classification system based on various specific agonists and their actions on biological systems, which respond to opioids. Around the mid 1960s it was proposed that more than one subtype of each major group of opioid receptors would explain some of the responses of receptors to multiple ligands. An example of this is the differences in respiratory depression caused by various MOP agonists. More recently, these data have been brought into question by the discovery that animals lacking genes coding a single variant of the Mu receptor lack any of the expected MOP responses, implying that the receptor systems do not work the way we currently believe them to. Research into the mechanisms of receptor function is ongoing and the current model is likely to change before long.

The most up-to-date classification of opioid receptors, their ligands and actions is that published by the International Union of Basic and Clinical Pharmacology (IUPHAR), which lists four types of receptors, MOP, DOP, KOP and NOP. MOP receptors are broken into Mu1, Mu2 and M3. Mu 1 and 2 are found in nervous tissue in the brain, spinal cord and

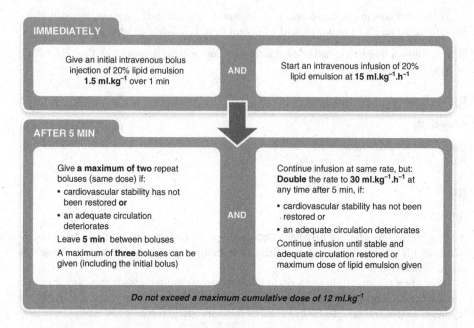

IMMEDIATELY

Give an initial intravenous bolus injection of 20% lipid emulsion **1.5 ml.kg^{-1}** over 1 min

AND

Start an intravenous infusion of 20% lipid emulsion at **15 ml.kg^{-1}.h^{-1}**

AFTER 5 MIN

Give **a maximum of two** repeat boluses (same dose) if:
- cardiovascular stability has not been restored **or**
- an adequate circulation deteriorates

Leave **5 min** between boluses

A maximum of **three** boluses can be given (including the initial bolus)

AND

Continue infusion at same rate, but: **Double** the rate to **30 ml.kg^{-1}.h^{-1}** at any time after 5 min, if:
- cardiovascular stability has not been restored or
- an adequate circulation deteriorates

Continue infusion until stable and adequate circulation restored or maximum dose of lipid emulsion given

Do not exceed a maximum cumulative dose of 12 ml.kg^{-1}

An approximate dose regimen for a 70-kg patient would be as follows:

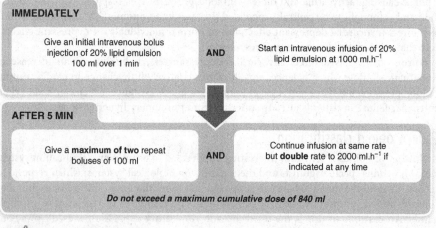

IMMEDIATELY

Give an initial intravenous bolus injection of 20% lipid emulsion 100 ml over 1 min

AND

Start an intravenous infusion of 20% lipid emulsion at 1000 ml.h^{-1}

AFTER 5 MIN

Give a **maximum of two** repeat boluses of 100 ml

AND

Continue infusion at same rate but **double** rate to 2000 ml.h^{-1} if indicated at any time

Do not exceed a maximum cumulative dose of 840 ml

This AAGBI Safety Guideline was produced by a Working Party that comprised:
Grant Cave, Will Harrop-Griffiths (Chair), Martyn Harvey, Tim Meek, John Picard, Tim Short and Guy Weinberg.
This Safety Guideline is endorsed by the Australian and New Zealand College of Anaesthetists (ANZCA).

Fig. B8. AAGBI Safety Guideline. *Management of Severe Local Anaesthetic Toxicity* (reproduced with permission from © The Association of Anaesthetists of Great Britain and Ireland 2010).

periphery. Mu1 agonists are mainly analgesic, Mu2 are analgesic, but also give rise to GI, respiratory and cutaneous effects (pruritus). Mu3 have various roles, including modulation of the immune system via the release of NO. DOP receptors are subclassified into Delta 1 and Delta 2. Both have roles in analgesia and are thought to be cardioprotective. Delta 2 receptors are part of the thermoregulatory system and are found in the brain and spinal cord. Delta 1 receptors are found in the brain and periphery but not in the spinal cord. The KOP group includes five receptors. Kappa1alpha and beta, Kappa2 alpha and beta and Kappa3. Kappa1alpha receptors are found in the nucleus accumbens. Kappa1beta are found in the neocortex and cerebellum. Both are analgesic and are thought to have roles in appetite regulation. Kappa2alpha receptors are found throughout the brain, Kappa2beta are found in the hippocampus, thalamus and brainstem. Both are analgesic and have neuroendocrine roles including fluid balance. Kappa3 receptors are found in the brain, but their action is poorly defined. NOP receptors are not yet linked with any agonists and are therefore not broken down into pharmacological subgroups like the other three groups. It is thought that periaqueductal grey matter contains NOP receptors, but work is ongoing in this area. Receptors with no known ligands are known as orphan receptors and the NOP receptor is an example of this.

Scott T, Swanevelder J. Perioperative myocardial protection. *Contin Educ Anaesth Crit Care Pain* 2009; **9**(3): 97–101

B10

Answer: a.

Non-specific low back pain refers to back pain with symptoms such as stiffness and soreness for which it is not possible to find a cause of the pain. The National Institute for Health and Clinical Excellence (NICE) issued guidelines in 2009 relating to the management of non-specific lower back pain of between 6 weeks' and 12 months' duration. Their guidelines were as follows:

- Offer one of the following:
  - A structured exercise programme tailored to the person
  - A course of manual therapy, e.g. spinal manipulation
  - Acupuncture
- Offer a combined physical and psychological treatment programme for those who have received the above, or have a greater disability
- Refer for possible spinal fusion if pain still severe

The use of imaging in the absence of red flags is inappropriate as would be starting an anti-neuropathic pain medication.

National Institute for Health and Clinical Excellence. Low back pain. Early management of persistent non-specific low back pain. Clinical guideline 88. Issue date: May 2009

B11

Answer: c.

ICS indications include:

- Anticipated blood loss of >1000 ml or >20% estimated blood volume
- Patients with a low Hb or increased risk factors for bleeding

- Patients with multiple antibodies or rare blood types
- Patients with objections to receiving allogeneic (donor) blood

ICS has been approved for use in urological malignancies. There are no proven cases of amniotic fluid embolus as a result of ICS and so it has been approved by NICE in obstetrics. Substances that should not be aspirated into the ICS system include: antibiotics not licensed for iv use; iodine; topical clotting agents; orthopaedic cement.

Some Jehovah's witnesses will accept salvaged blood.

The Association of Anaesthetists of Great Britain and Northern Ireland. Blood transfusion and the anaesthetist: intra-operative cell salvage. September 2009

B12

Answer: d.

Acromegaly is caused by secretion of growth hormone from eosinophil tumours of the anterior pituitary. If this occurs before fusion of the epiphysial plates, then the result is gigantism. Some cases are also caused by ectopic growth hormone secretion, but this is very rare. Altogether, acromegaly has an incidence of 6–8 per million per year.

Acromegaly tends to be associated with hyperglycaemia. This should be controlled with sliding scale insulin if necessary. Many of these patients suffer with diabetes mellitus and their glucose control should be assessed preoperatively.

Upper airway obstruction may result from macrognathia, macroglossia, hypertrophy of pharyngeal tissues, epiglottic hypertrophy and narrowing of the laryngeal lumen. Maintaining a patent airway can be challenging as can intubation. These patients are at increased risk of sleep apnoea and must be carefully observed postoperatively.

Both thyroid and adrenal function may be impaired due to decreased TSH and ACTH production in the pituitary. Patients may require assessment by an endocrinologist preoperatively to ensure they are as close to euthyroid as possible and to optimize their steroid treatment.

Seidman PA. Anaesthetic complications of acromegaly. *Br J Anaesth* 2000; **84**(2): 179–182

B13

Answer: c.

Anterograde cardioplegia is delivered by pumping the solution into the aortic root proximal to the cross clamp. It requires a competent aortic valve to prevent LV dilation and to ensure the fluid perfuses the coronary arteries. Retrograde delivery can be accomplished without a fully functional aortic valve, but cardiac arrest is less rapid. Cold cardioplegia solutions are associated with greater reperfusion injury, but warm solutions are associated with warm ischaemic injury if flow is intermittent. A compromise in this situation is to use warm solution to achieve arrest and then use cold solution intermittently. Cardioplegia requires around 20 mmol/l of potassium to achieve cardiac arrest and should be slightly hyperosmolar to prevent myocardial oedema.

Scott T, Swanevelder J., Perioperative myocardial protection. *Contin Educ Anaesth Crit Care Pain* 2009; **9**(3): 97–101

B14

Answer: a.

Preoperative hypotension and hypovolaemia in combination with renal ischaemia from aortic cross-clamping increases the risk of postoperative renal impairment. There is no strong evidence to suggest that any of the mentioned strategies have any benefit to renal function above the maintenance of an adequate extracellular volume and adequate perfusion pressure.

Leonard A. Anaesthesia for ruptured aortic aneurysm. *CEACCP* 2008; 8(1): 11–15

B15

Answer: d.

Pain and postoperative residual curarization would not account for the pyrexia, and malignant hyperthermia is characterized by muscle rigidity. This is most likely a thyroid storm, which usually occurs 6–24 hours postoperatively, but can occur sooner or intraoperatively.

Malhotra S, Sodhi V. Anaesthesia for thyroid and parathyroid surgery. *Contin Educ Anaesth Crit Care Pain* 2007; 7(2): 55–58

B16

Answer: d.

Primary haemorrhage after tonsillectomy is due to failure of haemostasis. It usually occurs within 4 hours. It is generally venous in nature, but a large amount of blood may be lost before haemorrhage is recognized, particularly in relation to the total blood volume of the child. Most of the blood is swallowed and so assessment of hypovolaemia can be difficult. Secondary (delayed) haemorrhage suggests infection. The role of NSAIDs has not been established, but it is unlikely to be significant and indeed some authors recommend 'liberal use of NSAIDs'.

Intubation of a patient with a primary haemorrhage after tonsillectomy can be challenging, even if their first intubation was straightforward. Pharyngeal trauma may be evident from the first intubation. Laryngeal oedema may be caused by the insertion of the previous endotracheal tube. Blood in the oropharynx is never the anaesthetist's friend!

The danger of pulmonary aspiration of regurgitated swallowed blood must be borne in mind. To this end, some recommend rapid sequence induction. The danger of regurgitation must be balanced against the possibility of cardiovascular collapse on induction as hypovolaemia is unmasked. The increased difficulty of intubation at the second anaesthetic may also be of concern if rapid sequence induction is to be employed, particularly since proper preoxygenation is difficult in an anxious child. If these problems are thought potentially significant, then gas induction in the left lateral position is permissible using sevoflurane in oxygen. It is important not to over-anaesthetize the patient during a gas induction, and it my be difficult to intubate while the patient is on their side.

However one proceeds, it is vital that IV access and suction are readily available.

Brennan L, Prabhu A. Paediatric day case anaesthesia. *Contin Educ Anaesth Crit Care Pain* 2003; 3(5): 134–138
Ravi R, Howell T. Anaesthesia for paediatric ear nose and throat surgery. *Contin Educ Anaesth Crit Care Pain* 2007; 7(2): 33–37

B17

Answer: a.

von Willebrand's disease is inherited in an autosomal dominant manner. It is the commonest inherited bleeding disorder. Typical symptoms include mucosal bleeding, easy bruising and menorrhagia. Platelet count is typically normal, the bleeding time is increased and factor VIII activity is often reduced.

von Willebrand's factor (vWF) is stored in platelets and acts as an adhesive bridge between platelets and damaged subendothelium at the site of vascular injury (primary haemostasis). It also functions as the carrier protein for factor VIII and as such is also involved in secondary haemostasis.

There are three main types: Type 1 (most common) has reduced amount of a functionally normal vWF. Symptoms are usually mild. Type 2 is split into four subtypes (A, B, M and N). Type 3 (least common) is the most severe form.

Datta, S. (ed.) Chapter 22: in *Hematologic Disease, Anaesthetic and Obstetric Management of High-Risk Pregnancy, 3rd edn*, 2004. *New York: Springer*

B18

Answer: a.

The anhepatic phase begins when the native liver is excised. It ends when venous clamps are released and the new donor liver is perfused. During this phase, the large citrate load from blood products cannot be metabolized, leading to hypocalcaemia. Myocardial depression occurs secondary to this. While a low cardiac output occurs, overzealous fluid administration may result in an engorged liver and intestines, making the surgery technically more difficult during the reperfusion phase. Acidaemia, not alkalaemia, occurs during the anhepatic phase.

Steadman R. Anaesthesia for liver transplant surgery. *Anaesthesiol Clin N Am* 2004; **22**: 687–711

Morgan GE, Mikhail MS. *Clinical Anaesthesiology* 4th edn, 2006. USA: McGraw-Hill, 797–801

B19

Answer: d.

Red flags are potential serious organic causes of back pain, which must be ruled out before embarking on standard mechanical lower back pain management. These red flags are:

- Presentation <20 or >55 years old
- Constant, progressive non-mechanical pain
- Past history of cancer, steroids, HIV, intravenous drug abuse
- Weight loss or systemically unwell
- Violent trauma
- Thoracic pain
- Widespread neurological symptoms/signs
- Structural deformity

- Cauda equina syndrome, suggested by sphincter disturbance, saddle anaesthesia and lower limb weakness

A history of intravenous drug use represents a red flag and should be investigated in this young woman to rule out a cause such as osteomyelitis. An MRI scan of her lumbar spine and routine blood tests should be done in the first instance. Once red flags are ruled out, an interdisciplinary approach is best adopted, including pharmacological, physical and psychological interventions.

Jackson MA, Simpson KH. Chronic back pain. *Contin Educ in Anaesth, Crit Care Pain* 2006;6 (4):152–155

Main CJ, Spanswick CC. *Pain Management – An Interdisciplinary Approach*, 1st edn, 2000. Edinburgh: Churchill Livingstone

B20
Answer: b.

It is essential candidates understand the physiology of the Fontan circulation and its relevance to anaesthesia.

Patients with a Fontan circulation have a passive circulation from venous system to pulmonary system. It is important to ensure that the patient does not become bradycardic or hypotensive and to reduce any increase in pulmonary vascular resistance. Nausea and vomiting may be symptoms of hypoperfusion. It is important to ensure the physiological parameters are maintained within normal limits for this patient. Although spontaneous ventilation is preferred, in this scenario, it is important to ensure she does not aspirate.

Nayak S, Booker P. The Fontan circulation. *Contin Educ Anaesth Crit Care Pain* 2008; 8(1): 26–30

B21
Answer: d.

ARDS is the severe form of ALI. The diagnostic criteria for ALI are as follows:

- Acute onset
- Bilateral diffuse infiltrates on CXR
- Pulmonary wedge pressure ≤18 mmHg or absence of clinical evidence of left atrial hypertension
- Hypoxaemia with $P_aO_2/F_IO_2 < 40\,kPa$

The diagnostic criteria for ARDS differ from ALI only in the P_aO_2/F_IO_2 ratio; $< 27\,kPa$.

Of those patients ventilated in critical care, approximately 16% will develop ALI. This may be a reflection of the severity of the underlying pathology, but ALI may in itself contribute to organ failure. Rates of mortality and morbidity are high.

Causes of ALI can be classified as either *direct* (an insult to the lung cells) or *indirect* (a result of an acute inflammatory response). The most common cause is sepsis, other causes are listed below:

- Direct – pneumonia, aspiration, smoke inhalation, pulmonary embolism
- Indirect – sepsis, pancreatitis, blood transfusion, trauma, burns

The pathophysiological course is similar for ALI and ARDS and is irrespective of the cause. Three overlapping phases are described.

1. Acute or exudative phase: characterized by hypoxaemia, infiltrates on CXR and reduced lung compliance
2. Subacute or proliferative phase: characterized by persistent hypoxaemia, increased dead space and reduced compliance
3. Chronic or fibrotic phase: resulting from pulmonary fibrosis and leading to loss of normal lung structure

Ventilatory strategies are designed to reduce barotrauma and are based on avoiding large lung volumes and peak pressures.

Mackay A, Al-Haddad M. Acute lung injury and acute respiratory distress syndrome. *Contin Educ Anaesth Crit Care Pain* 2009; **9**(5): 152–156

B22

Answer: c.

Dementia is a cognitive impairment developing slowly over a number of years. In contrast, delirium is an acutely developing cognitive impairment together with a change in consciousness. It can be either hyper- or hypoactive in nature. The hypoactive forms are easily missed. Any form of dementia can co-exist with any other psychiatric disorder and this can make diagnosis and treatment very challenging. In patients who require treatment, the first-line therapy is haloperidol. In patients who cannot tolerate haloperidol, for example, those with long QT syndrome who are at risk of torsades, the treatment of choice is olanzepine. Benzodiazepines have a strong association with delirium and can worsen symptoms. Smoking is one of several patient risk factors for delirium in the ICU. Others include alcohol misuse, pre-existing cognitive dysfunction and increasing age. Sleep disturbance is a major healthcare-related factor and illness-related factors include anaemia, hypotension and metabolic disturbances, which need not be profound to cause significant delirium. Delirium is often misdiagnosed as some form of psychosis particularly when the delirium involves hallucinations and delusions. Delirious patients tend to have visual hallucinations accompanied by a change in consciousness, whereas schizophrenic patients tend to have auditory hallucinations and there is not necessarily a change in consciousness.

Fines DP, Severn AM. Anaesthesia and cognitive disturbance in the elderly. *Contin Educ Anaesth Crit Care Pain* 2006; **6**(1):37–40

B23

Answer: a.

More hydrophilic opioids have a tendency to spread cephalad and cause late-onset respiratory depression. Fentanyl is the least hydrophilic and causes the least depression. Diamorphine is partially metabolized *in situ*, giving a useful compromise between lipophilicity and duration of action. Recent NICE guidance suggests that 0.3–0.4 mg of diamorphine should be used in intrathecal blocks in place of the 20–30 μg of fentanyl that had been previously used. All opioids, including the phenylpiperidine derivatives, are associated with pruritus. This is especially troublesome in obstetrics for reasons which are not well understood.

Morphine is very hydrophilic and binds very poorly to non-receptor sites such as myelin. This is in contrast to more lipophilic drugs such as fentanyl. The result is that morphine has a very low volume of distribution within the CSF and an accompanying increase in the likelihood of late-onset respiratory depression even at low doses.

Hindle A. Intrathecal opioids in the management of acute postoperative pain. *Contin Educ Anaesth Crit Care Pain* 2008; 8(3): 81–85

B24

Answer: b.

Knowledge of resuscitation algorithms is important for the FRCA. This question tests knowledge of the status epilepticus algorithm contained in the Advanced Paediatric Life Support Course. The question is structured this way because questions regarding algorithms (ALS, APLS, AAGBI, etc.) do exist and will only be passed if the correct path is followed.

Key aspects of this algorithm:

- As with all paediatric emergencies: assess/open the airway, give oxygen, don't forget glucose
- The first-line treatment is a benzodiazepine
- Up to 5 minutes is permitted from the start of the convulsion to gain vascular access (iv/io). If successful: lorazepam 0.1 mg/kg
- If vascular access fails, use alternative routes (rectal – diazepam, 0.5 mg/kg, buccal – midazolam, 0.1 mg/kg)
- Allow 10 minutes for benzodiazepines to work. Re-attempt vascular access during this time if not secured. If seizure activity continues, call for senior help and give iv/io lorazepam (0.1 mg/kg). Calling for senior help before this is not wrong.
- Give iv/io lorazepam
- Wait 10 minutes
- Give second-line drug: phenytoin 20 mg/kg (unless already on phenytoin, then give phenobarbitone 20 mg/kg
- Wait 20 minutes
- Perform RSI with thiopentone (anaesthetist must be present by this stage)

Chapter 12 – The convulsing child, in *Advanced Paediatric Life Support Manual* 5th edn, 2011. Wiley-Blackwell. 128–135

B25

Answer: d.

Most patients with sickle cell disease have a chronically low Hb and the above situation may not necessitate a transfusion. Ideally, the case should be discussed with a haematologist. Any of the answers could possibly be correct. However, TRALI and acute haemolytic reactions are rare, sickle chest syndrome commonly presents with chest pain, and fat embolism would also be unlikely from a humeral fracture.

TRALI is a rare complication of blood transfusion, and complicates one in many thousands of transfusions (incidence varies between countries and between blood components). It is unusual among immune reactions to blood; the physiological response is thought to be mediated by donor leukocytes attacking pulmonary endothelium, rather than a host response to foreign antigens. The clinical presentation resembles the familiar syndromes of ALI/ARDS encountered in critical care, and presents a short number of hours after commencement of transfusion with tachycardia, dyspnoea, cyanosis, acute hypoxaemia and, sometimes, hypotension.

Acute haemolytic reactions are usually releated to ABO or other surface antigen incompatibility, and occasionally due to transfusion of damaged red cells. Reactions can be fatal, and complicate 1 : 6000 – 1 : 33000 transfusions. There is severe intravascular haemolysis, associated with coagulopathy and haematuria.

Acute sickle chest syndrome is an important complication of sickle cell disease, and is one type of sickle cell crisis. Vascular occlusion in the pulmonary circulation results in fever, cough and chest pain. In North America it is the second commonest cause of hospital admission in sickle cell patients, and is responsible for 25% of deaths.

Fat embolism syndrome (FES) is most commonly associated with long bone and pelvic fractures. The incidence following a single long bone fracture is 1%–3%, but increases to 33% of patients with bilateral femoral fractures. Non-trauma causes include pancreatitis and sickle cell crisis. FES is classically described as a triad of respiratory changes (tachypnoea, dyspnoea, hypoxaemia) neurological abnormalities (acute confusion, seizures) and petechial rash (especially of the upper body, oral mucosa and conjunctivae).

Gupta A, Reilly C. Fat embolism. *Contin Educ Anaesth Crit Care Pain* 2007; 5: 148–151
Silliman CC, Ambruso DR, Boshkov LK. Transfusion-related acute lung injury. *Blood* 2005; 105: 2266–2273

B26

Answer: b.

This patient has rhabdomyolysis and acute renal failure. Goal-directed fluid resuscitation with non-potassium containing fluids is vital as hypovolaemia worsens any renal damage caused by myoglobin. Alkalinization of the urine will help as it increases the solubility of the Tamm–Horsfall protein (THP) and myoglobin complex. Urinary pH should be maintained at levels >7. Diuretics can be used, but it is controversial. Despite treatment, ARF can occur and renal replacement therapy is indicated if there is persisting oliguria and metabolic abnormalities.

Hunter JD, Gregg K, Damani Z. Rhabdomyolysis. *Contin Educ Anaesth Crit Care Pain* 2006; 6: 141–143

B27

Answer: b.

Neuropathic pain arises from a heterogeneous group of disorders that affect the peripheral and central nervous systems. Some common examples include painful diabetic neuropathy, postherpetic and trigeminal neuralgia. Neuropathic pain is often difficult to treat as it is resistant to many medications or because of the adverse effects associated with effective medications. Drugs used to manage neuropathic pain include: antidepressants, anticonvulsant drugs, opioids and topical treatments such as capsaicin and lidocaine. NICE guidelines published in March 2010 have recommended the following in the management of neuro-pathic pain in the non-specialist setting:

First-line treatment

In non-diabetic neuropathy the use of oral amitriptyline or pregabalin is indicated. For those individuals who have benefited from amitriptyline as first-line treatment, but cannot tolerate the adverse effects, either oral imipramine or nortriptyline can be considered as alternatives. For painful diabetic neuropathy, oral duloxetine is the first-line treatment.

Second-line treatment

If first-line treatment was with amitriptyline, switch to or combine with oral pregabalin. If first-line treatment was with pregabalin, switch to or combine with oral amitriptyline.

Third-line treatment

Refer to specialist pain service and consider oral tramadol alone or in combination with the second-line treatment. Topical lidocaine can also be considered when oral medications cannot be tolerated.

NICE Clinical guideline 96. Neuropathic pain – the pharmacological management of neuropathic pain in adults in non-specialist settings. Accessed from: www.nice.org.uk/guidance/CG96, 2010

B28

Answer: c.

Neurogenic diabetes insipidus (DI) is associated with traumatic brain injury (incidence up to 35%), subarachnoid haemorrhage and pituitary surgery. Development of DI following non-pituitary surgery is often associated with severe cerebral oedema. DI may be transient or permanent. It occurs as a result of failure of ADH release from the hypothalamic–pituitary axis. This leads to the production of large volumes of dilute urine (as the body is unable to concentrate the urine) and inappropriate loss of water. The patient becomes clinically dehydrated and hypernatraemic. Typically, patients may have a urine output >6 l day^{-1}. Consider other causes of polyuria in neurosurgical patients, e.g. osmotic diuretics, intra-venous fluid administration, hypertonic saline and triple-H therapy (used to treat cerebral vasospasm). The raised creatinine would not be specific to DI.

The conscious patient will complain of polyuria, polydipsia and thirst. Hyperglycaemia should be excluded as a cause. In the context of brain injury, the diagnosis of DI is made in the presence of:

- Increased urine volume (usually >3000 ml per 24 h)
- High serum sodium (>145 mmol/l)
- High serum osmolality (>305 mmol/kg)
- Abnormally low urine osmolality (<350 mmol/kg)
- Urine specific gravity <1.005 in presence of other features is suggestive (useful bedside test)

The management of DI is to replace the water deficit and to replace ADH. If urine output continues >250 ml per hour, synthetic ADH should be administered; this is usually in the form of intranasal DDAVP 100–200 mcg or as an intravenous dose (0.4 mcg).

Bradshaw K, Smith M. Disorders of sodium balance after brain injury. *Contin Educ Anaesth Crit Care Pain* 2008; **8**(4): 129–133

B29

Answer: d.

In 2001 Rafi described palpating the triangle of Petit, which can be found below the costal margin, above the iliac crest and between the lattisimus dorsi and the external oblique. The triangle is felt as a 'dimple' under the skin and represents the point of minimal thickness of the abdominal wall. If the block is performed here, only one 'pop' will be felt as the external oblique is not pierced. The block is performed with a short needle, which may be blunted to increase the 'pop' sensation on crossing layers of the abdominal wall. A longer needle risks piercing the peritoneum or damaging abdominal organs. It is unlikely that the block will extend further than T10 – L1 with a single injection. It is possible to augment the block with a second subcostal injection.

In an adult 20 ml of 0.5% bupivacaine is required for each side to provide a reliable block. This would be equal to 200 mg of bupivacaine, which would be above the recommended maximum dose for a patient weighing 70 kg.

Mukhtar K. Transversus abdominis plane block. *J N Y School Regional Anaesth* 2009; **12**:28–33.
Rafi A. Abdominal field block: a new approach via the lumbar triangle. *Anaesthesia* 2001; **56**:1024–1026

B30

Answer: a.

The majority of cases of acute asthma will respond adequately to bolus nebulization of β_2 agonists; with the use of continuous nebulization of β_2 agonists indicated for those patients with a poor response to initial bolus therapy.

Inhaled β_2 agonists are as efficacious as and preferable to intravenous β_2 agonists, with the latter being reserved for those circumstances where the inhaled route cannot be reliably used. The combination of parental β_2 agonists and inhaled β_2 agonists may have a role in ventilated patients or those in extremis.

The use of adrenaline is not recommended as it does not have significant benefit over salbutamol or terbutaline.

British Guideline in the Management of Asthma. *A National Clinical Guideline*, 2011. London: British Thoracic Society.

Paper C – Questions

C1

Sedation and anaesthesia are often required to enable dental treatment to be performed.

Concerning the following statements regarding dental procedures, which is most accurate?
a. General anaesthesia for dental treatment may only be provided outside the hospital setting by a consultant anaesthetist and operating department practitioner
b. A mix of nitrous oxide 60% and oxygen 40% is commonly used as inhaled sedation for paediatric patients
c. Intravenous conscious sedation may be administered by appropriately trained dental practitioners
d. Propofol administered as a target-controlled infusion should be avoided due to the possibility of impaired airway reflexes in a shared airway
e. Intravenous access is not mandatory during inhalational anaesthesia for very short procedures in children

C2

The major factor responsible for the spread of particles, including micro-organisms, by anaesthetists in the operating theatre is:
a. Failure to wear an appropriate facemask
b. Wearing scrub clothing laundered at home
c. Entering and leaving the operating theatre
d. Failing to don sterile gloves for insertion of iv cannulae
e. Carrying a briefcase and/or backpack into the operating theatre

C3

A 35-year-old female requires a vaginal hysterectomy for menorrhagia. The patient plays competitive tennis and has a body mass index of 38 kg/m^2. The expected duration of surgery is 70 minutes.

Appropriate perioperative thromboprophylaxis for this patient would be graduated compression stockings and:
a. Early mobilization
b. Aspirin 150 mg daily commenced 12 hours preoperatively

Practice Single Best Answer Questions for the Final FRCA, ed. Hozefa Ebrahim, Khalid Hasan, Mark Tindall, Michael Clarke and Natish Bindal. Published by Cambridge University Press. © Cambridge University Press 2013.

49

c. Enoxaparin 0.5 mg/kg daily commenced within 6 hours of surgery
d. Enoxaparin 0.5 mg/kg daily commenced 12 hours preoperatively
e. Full leg sequential compression device

C4

You have been asked to anaesthetize a 72-year-old man for an emergency MRI scan of the lumbar spine to rule out spinal cord compression.

Which of the following is the most valid consideration?
a. The use of 100% inspired oxygen should be reported to the radiologist as it may cause degradation of the images
b. You must wear ear protection in the scanning room if the noise level produced exceeds 90 dB
c. Gadolinium-based contrast agents should be avoided due to the relatively high incidence of allergic reactions
d. The presence of a modern spinal cord neurostimulator should pose little risk in a 1.5-T scanner
e. Quenching of the magnet in an emergency situation will result in a hypoxic environment in the scan room

C5

An 80-year-old woman is referred to the ICU. She had developed acute renal failure and had become profoundly hypotensive with a mean arterial pressure of 40 mmHg. She has been treated for a urinary tract infection. Blood cultures are positive for Gram-positive bacteria.

The most likely organism from the following list given the history is:
a. *Staphylococcus saprophyticus*
b. *Proteus mirabilis*
c. *Enterococcus faecalis*
d. *Candida albicans*
e. *Escherichia coli*

C6

Regional anaesthesia can be used to avoid the risks of general anaesthesia, but is not without risks of its own.

Which of the following is true?
a. Bupivacaine has greater α_1-adrenoceptor activity than other local anaesthetics
b. If lipid emulsion is not available, then a propofol infusion can be used instead for bupivacaine toxicity
c. Addition of adrenaline doubles the safe dose of bupivacaine
d. High cardiac output states reduce the likelihood of local anaesthetic toxicity
e. Lipid emulsions are of no use in the treatment of lidocaine toxicity

C7

Guillain–Barré syndrome (GBS) is an acute inflammatory polyneuropathy first described in the latter half of the nineteenth century.

Regarding GBS:
a. Suxamethonium is contraindicated because GBS is a demyelinating upper motor neurone disease
b. Around 30% of GBS patients require respiratory support
c. If onset is rapid, then recovery is generally also rapid
d. Paraesthesia is not a common feature
e. Autonomic dysfunction is uncommon, with motor dysfunction being the primary problem

C8

A 32-year-old man has undergone a recent traumatic amputation of his left forearm. Shortly before his discharge from hospital, he reports painful, unpleasant sensations in the distribution of the amputated limb. In particular, he is troubled by the sensation of involuntary spasms.

Which of the following actions would you undertake first?
a. Arrange a prescription of regular oral NSAIDs
b. Arrange TENS therapy
c. Refer the patient for a course of acupuncture
d. Arrange mirror-box therapy
e. Refer for consideration for spinal cord stimulation (SCS)

C9

A 70-kg man is admitted to neuro-critical care with a diffuse axonal head injury following a road traffic collision. He is intubated and ventilated. He is being enterally fed via a nasogastric tube.

Which of the following statements most accurately describes his daily nutritional requirements?
a. Water 1200 ml, glucose 70 g, protein 35 g, phosphate 10 mmol
b. Water 2500 ml, glucose 140 g, protein 70 g, phosphate 30 mmol
c. Water 2500 ml, glucose 140 g, protein 140 g, phosphate 60 mmol
d. Water 2100 ml, glucose 70 g, protein 35 g, potassium 30 mmol
e. Water 1200 ml, glucose 140 g, protein 140 g, potassium 10 mmol

C10

A surgeon wants to infiltrate an open appendicectomy wound with some local anaesthetic. The patient, a 6-year-old, 18-kg child has had no other local anaesthetic.

What is the safe maximum dose of bupivacaine for this child?
a. 3 ml of 0.5% levobupivicaine
b. 7 ml of 0.5% bupivacaine
c. 13 ml of 0.75% ropivacaine
d. 10 ml of 0.375% ropivacaine with adrenaline 1:200 000
e. 20 ml of 0.25% bupivacaine with adrenaline 1:200 000

C11

A 78-year-old man presents for a hernia repair. During his preoperative assessment he tells the anaesthesiologist he has episodic stabbing pain in his right foot precipitated by pressure.

51

There are no sensory, motor or excretory deficits. He requests anaesthetic advice on therapy. He has been taking paracetamol to little effect.

What would be the most appropriate initial therapy while awaiting assessment at the pain clinic?

a. Duloxetine
b. Carbamazepine
c. Amitriptyline
d. Gabapentin
e. Codeine

C12

A 26-year-old gentleman is admitted to the emergency department with a closed traumatic brain injury following a road traffic collision. On application of a painful central stimulus, his eyes remain closed, he extends his left arm and he makes incomprehensible sounds. Computed tomography (CT) of the head reveals a large left-sided fronto-parietal contusion with obvious midline shift.

Which of the following would be the most appropriate initial interventions, after intubation and ventilation?

a. Aim for a P_aCO_2 of 4.5 kPa, maintenance of a mean arterial pressure of 80 mmHg, and active cooling to a core temperature of 34 °C
b. Aim for a P_aCO_2 of 4.5 kPa, insertion of an intracranial pressure monitor and maintenance of a cerebral perfusion pressure of 60 mmHg
c. Aim for a P_aCO_2 of 4.5 kPa and maintenance of a mean arterial pressure of 100 mmHg
d. Aim for a P_aCO_2 of 4.0 kPa and maintenance of a mean arterial pressure of 80 mmHg
e. Aim for a P_aCO_2 of 4.5 kPa, maintenance of a mean arterial pressure of 80 mmHg and administration of high-dose intravenous methylprednisolone

C13

A hypotensive 20-year-old man in intensive care was diagnosed to have acute renal dysfunction secondary to rhabdomyolysis after being involved in a road traffic accident. He was initially treated with aggressive fluid therapy and diuretics.

Which is the most appropriate drug to be started in order to maintain adequate renal perfusion?

a. Vasopressin
b. Dopamine
c. Adrenaline
d. Noradrenaline
e. Mannitol

C14

A previously fit and well 3-year-old girl is brought into hospital by her parents with a 1-day history of being unwell, pyrexial and suffering right iliac fossa pain. She is listed by the surgeons for an appendicectomy. During the operation, she is found to have an inflamed appendix and localized peritonitis. At the end of the procedure, the surgeon infiltrates local anaesthetic around the wound edges.

The most appropriate postoperative pain relief would be:
a. Regular paracetamol and ibuprofen
b. Regular paracetamol, ibuprofen and patient-controlled morphine analgesia (PCA)
c. Regular paracetamol, ibuprofen and nurse-controlled morphine analgesia (NCA)
d. Regular paracetamol, ibuprofen and a continuous morphine infusion
e. Regular paracetamol, ibuprofen and Oramorph PRN

C15

A 35-year-old woman with gallstone pancreatitis is ventilated on ICU. Her chest X-ray shows bilateral infiltrates and her arterial blood gas shows a p_aO_2 7 kPa on a F_iO_2 1.0. You diagnose her with acute respiratory distress syndrome (ARDS).

Which of the following interventions has been shown to reduce mortality in ARDS?
a. Intravenous methylprednisolone
b. Inhaled nitric oxide
c. Ventilation with 6 ml/kg tidal volumes
d. Prone positioning
e. Intravenous furosemide infusion

C16

An extremely anxious 27-year-old female is listed for an urgent laparoscopic cholecystectomy. She is currently on methadone, having abused opioids in the past. Problems with pain control following her last operation are documented.

Which preoperative intervention is most likely to reduce postoperative pain problems this time?
a. Patient reassurance
b. 8 mg iv dexamethasone
c. 100 mg oral diclofenac and 2 g oral paracetamol
d. 600 mg oral gabapentin
e. 20 mg oral temazepam

C17

The incidence and prevalence of liver disease is increasing worldwide.

What is the most common cause of acute hepatic failure in the UK?
a. Ethanol
b. 3, 4-methylenedioxymethamphetamine
c. *Amanita phalloides*
d. Viral hepatitis
e. Acetaminophen

C18

You are asked to assess a patient in the obstetric clinic who has von Willebrand's disease. She is keen to have an epidural for labour if required. There are several types of this disease.

Which type of von Willebrand's disease commonly worsens during pregnancy?
a. Type 1
b. Type 2A
c. Type 2B

d. Type 2M

e. Type 3

C19

During the first few days of life, which of the following is the least likely to result in a transitional circulation?

a. Congenital diaphragmatic hernia

b. Necrotizing enterocolitis

c. Cardiac failure

d. Respiratory distress syndrome

e. Sepsis

C20

A 58-year-old woman with a 15-year history of rheumatoid arthritis is taking 160 mg of oral morphine per day.

Which of the following opioid patches would give her dose equivalence?

a. Buprenorphine 5 mcg/7days

b. Buprenorphine 10 mcg/7days

c. Fentanyl 25 mcg/72 hours

d. Fentanyl 50 mcg/72 hrs

e. Fentanyl 75 mcg/72 hrs

C21

Whilst on your preoperative visit a patient informs you they are taking St John's Wort (SJW) as well as their normal medications.

Which of the following statements is false?

a. SJW is used by patients for the treatment of mood disorders

b. SJW can cause an accumulation of drugs such as warfarin

c. SJW can cause severe autonomic dysfunction in some patients

d. SJW should ideally be paused 5 days or more before surgery

e. SJW can cause prolonged sedation after anaesthesia

C22

A 28-year-old woman of 32 weeks' gestation is admitted to the labour ward from triage with hypertension, headache and epigastric pain. She is not in labour. Her vital signs are: blood pressure 170/109, heart rate 100 bpm, 3^+ proteinuria on dipstick. She has two beats of ankle clonus. The fetal heart rate is reassuring. She has not received any medication.

What would you do next?

a. Administer labetalol 100 mg orally

b. Administer magnesium sulphate 4 g iv bolus followed by infusion

c. Arrange for urgent Caesarean section

d. Commence hydralazine infusion iv

e. Administer nifedipine 20 mg orally

C23

You are anaesthetizing a 4-year-old child for unilateral squint correction. The child is breathing spontaneously on sevoflurane. Her heart rate drops to 40 bpm.

Which of the following is correct?
a. Hypocarbia increases the incidence of significant bradycardia
b. She is at increased risk of postoperative nausea and vomiting
c. Oculocardiac reflex occurs in 90% of squint surgery cases
d. Oculocardiac reflex often results in major dysrhythmias
e. Oculocardiac reflex occurs most commonly when the lateral rectus muscle is manipulated

C24

You have anaesthetized a 64-year-old male for a left upper lobectomy for squamous cell carcinoma. You are currently ventilating both lungs and now want to test the tube position and proceed to deflate the left lung.

The first step you would take is:
a. Open the tracheal lumen and clamp the fresh gas flow to it
b. Inflate the bronchial cuff and confirm left-sided breath sounds
c. Use the fibre-optic scope to check the position of the tube
d. Open the bronchial lumen and clamp the fresh gas flow to it
e. Decrease by half the tidal volumes

C25

A 42-year-old motorcyclist is scheduled for a revision of a tibial plate to his lower left tibia as a result of misalignment. He requests a general anaesthetic and wants to be pain-free on awakening. The surgeons are keen for a regional block to allow him to mobilize early.

The best single block you could offer would be?
a. Lumbar plexus block
b. Lumbar epidural
c. 'Three in one' block
d. Posterior tibial block
e. Posterior sciatic block

C26

You have anaesthetized a 75-year-old patient for a below-knee amputation. The patient is diabetic with chronic renal failure on dialysis. There is significant blood loss intraoperatively requiring transfusion, and the surgeons are complaining 'he is very oozy'. Coagulation studies show platelets, PT, APTT and INR are normal, but bleeding time is prolonged.

The most appropriate management would be to:
a. Send the patient for immediate dialysis
b. Give cryoprecipitate

c. Give DDAVP 0.3 µg/kg
d. Give intravenous conjugated oestrogens
e. Give platelets

C27

A 35-year-old male with cystic fibrosis has had a bilateral sequential lung transplant and on day 1 postop has a falling cardiac output (CO) as measured by thermodilution technique using pulmonary artery catheter (PAC) measurements. Other findings include:

Temperature	37.8 °C
Heart rate	110 bpm paced rhythm (DDD mode)
Central venous pressure	23 cmH$_2$O
Pulmonary artery pressure (PAP)	34/22 mmHg

He is on nitric oxide, isoprenaline and noradrenaline.
The most likely reason for the fall in CO is
a. Acute rejection
b. Inappropriate pacemaker settings
c. Systemic inflammatory response syndrome (SIRS)
d. Right ventricular failure
e. Excessive nitric oxide administration

C28

You are about to anaesthetize a 60-year-old gentleman with moderate chronic obstructive airways disease for an elective laparotomy for a sigmoid tumour. You wish to site an epidural as part of your strategy for postoperative analgesia. The patient received a therapeutic dose of low-molecular-weight heparin 12 hours ago for a recent deep vein thrombosis.

What is the most appropriate step?
a. Continue with the case and site the epidural
b. Check the prothrombin time
c. Measure anti factor 10a levels
d. Postpone the case until at least another 12 hours have passed to site the epidural
e. Check the APTT ratio

C29

A 17-year-old, 65-kg male with Duchenne's muscular dystrophy requires a general anaesthetic for tonsillectomy. He is wheelchair-bound due to muscle weakness. His cough is good. His airway examination is unremarkable. He last ate 8 hours ago, and had clear fluids 4 hours ago.

Which is the most appropriate induction technique?
a. Rapid sequence iv induction with thiopentone, suxamethonium and cricoid pressure
b. Gas induction and use of non-depolarizing muscle relaxant in a reduced dose

c. Propofol + fentanyl induction, then use either suxamethonium or non-depolarizing muscle relaxants, but at approximately 20% of the normal dose
d. To use propofol TIVA and attempt intubation without muscle relaxants
e. Propofol + fentanyl induction, reduced dose of non-depolarizing muscle relaxant for intubation, then repeated dosing intraoperatively based on nerve stimulator activity

C30

A patient with obstructive sleep apnoea presents to your preoperative assessment clinic and you notice a polysomnography report in their notes.

Which of the following parameters is not routinely recorded during polysomnography?
a. Electroencephalogram
b. Oxygen saturations
c. End-tidal carbon dioxide
d. Electro-oculogram
e. Electromyogram

Paper C – Answers

C1

Answer: c.

A Department of Health report published in 2000 recommended that general anaesthesia for dental procedures must only be provided in a hospital setting by trained anaesthetists, following a number of deaths in dental practices where anaesthesia had been delivered. Dental practitioners with a qualification in conscious sedation may administer intravenous conscious sedation if strict guidelines are followed.

'Relative analgesia' using nitrous oxide and oxygen via a nasal mask is a safe and effective technique widely used in children. It is well tolerated and has a rapid recovery, but the concentration of nitrous oxide delivered should not exceed 30%.

Propofol TCI (target-controlled infusion) may be used by experienced anaesthetists in a hospital setting and results in a superior recovery profile compared to other techniques, but it is easy for the patient to lose control of their airway if the sedation depth increases, and therefore midazolam is usually the first-line choice of agent as it is easily titratable and rapidly reversible with flumazenil.

Intravenous access should be instigated even for short dental procedures as emergency agents such as suxamethonium and atropine may be required.

Conscious sedation in the provision of dental care. Report of an Expert Group on Sedation for Dentistry, Standing Dental Advisory Committee. DoH, London, 2003 (www.dh.gov.uk/en/Publicationsandstatistics/Publications/PublicationsPolicyAndGuidance/DH_4069257)

C2

Answer: c.

Facemasks are only required if the anaesthetist is a part of the operative field, particularly when inserting neuraxial blocks or central venous catheter. Scrubs may be laundered at home, but should only be donned in the operating theatre and must be changed daily. Entering and leaving the operating theatre generates air currents within the theatre and introduces particles and, potentially, organisms from outside the theatre. Sterile precautions while inserting intravenous cannula are essential to prevent infection in the patient

Practice Single Best Answer Questions for the Final FRCA, ed. Hozefa Ebrahim, Khalid Hasan, Mark Tindall, Michael Clarke and Natish Bindal. Published by Cambridge University Press. © Cambridge University Press 2013.

concerned, but do not contribute to the spread of particles. Briefcases and backpacks do not increase the risk of particle spread unless they are moved excessively.

Loftus RW, Koff MD, Burchman CC, *et al.* Transmission of pathogenic bacterial organisms in the anesthesia work area. *Anesthesiology* 2008; **109**: 399–407

C3

Answer: c.

The patient's BMI places her in an intermediate risk group as does the surgery she will undergo. Stockings, combined with early mobilization will be insufficient to substantially lower her risk of symptomatic postoperative venous thromboembolism and she requires pharmacological thromboprophylaxis. Enoxaparin is an appropriate agent. Given the risk of bleeding from pelvic surgery and the lack of evidence for a benefit from preoperative pharmacological prophylaxis, postoperative prophylaxis is the most appropriate intervention for this patient.

Davies RG, Rayment R. Primum non nocere – NICE guidelines on venous thromboembolism. *Anaesthesia* 2010; **65**(8): 774–778

C4

Answer: a.

The use of 100% inspired oxygen may indeed produce an artefact in the form of an abnormally high signal in the CSF in T2-weighted images. Ear protection must be used if the acoustic noise level exceeds 80 dB. Gadolinium-based contrast agents have the best safety profile of agents used to enhance the signal produced by tissues. They have a relatively low incidence of anaphylaxis (less than 1 in 100 000) and relatively mild side effects such as nausea, itching and urticaria (approximately 2%). They should not be used in patients with a glomerular filtration rate (GFR) of less than 30 ml/min as a potentially fatal condition known as nephrogenic systemic fibrosis may develop.

The presence of a neuro-stimulator is currently a contraindication for an MRI scan as thermal injury and equipment malfunction is likely.

Quenching the magnet is a disruptive and costly process and results in the sudden release of large quantities of helium from the superconductor magnet core. The helium should be vented away from the room, and an oxygen analyser is present in the room, which will alarm if a hypoxic environment is generated.

Safety in Magnetic Resonance Units 2010 – An Update. Association of Anaesthetists of Great Britain and Ireland. Guideline, 2010

C5

Answer: a.

The most likely causative organism from those listed is *Staphylococcus saprophyticus*. The Gram-negative organism *Escherichia coli* is the commonest cause of female urinary tract infections acquired in the community (80%–85%) followed by *Staphylococcus saprophyticus*, which is Gram-positive (10%). The other common organisms include *Klebsiella pneumonia* and *Proteus mirabilis*, which are both Gram-negative. In contrast,

Enterobacteriaciae are the commonest group of organisms in children. *Candida albicans* is a Gram-positive fungus.

Ronald A. The etiology of urinary tract infection: traditional and emerging pathogens. *Am J Med* 2002; **113**(1) S1: 14–19

C6

Answer: a.

Local anaesthetic toxicity is dangerous and carries a high mortality. Bupivacaine is particularly dangerous as it has a lower toxic dose than other agents and bupivacaine toxicity is resistant to treatment. Recent evidence shows that the use of lipid emulsions such as Intralipid ® can be of use during the resuscitation effort. Propofol is not a suitable substitute for lipid emulsions, but may be useful for controlling seizures if they occur. Addition of adrenaline does not change the toxic dose of bupivacaine, though it does alter doses of other local anaesthetics.

In the treatment of local anaesthetic toxicity, lipid emulsions work by binding the lipophilic local anaesthetic molecules. In doing this, they increase the volume of fat within which the drug is distributed and hence reduce its concentration. It has been said that lidocaine toxicity is not amenable to treatment with lipid emulsions because lidocaine is significantly less lipophilic than, for example, bupivacaine. This has been shown not to be the case and there are reports of successful resuscitation of patients after lidocaine overdoses, which had failed to respond to other treatments.

High cardiac output states increase the 'washout' of local anaesthetics from the tissues in which it is deposited. This has the effect of increasing plasma drug concentrations and therefore risk of toxicity.

Many local anaesthetics are direct myocardial depressants, but bupivacaine has a greater α_1 agonist action than, for example, ropivacaine and levobupivacaine. This is one reason why systemic toxicity is so difficult to treat. The combination of myocardial depression and increased afterload has been demonstrated both *in vitro* and *in vivo*. It has also been shown that the use of adrenaline in resuscitation efforts of local anaesthetic toxicity may be deleterious, prompting some to suggest that lipid emulsions, rather than being a treatment of last resort, should be a first-line response to this complication.

AAGBI Safety Guideline. *Management of Severe Local Anaesthetic Toxicity*, 2010

C7

Answer: b.

There are two forms of GBS, demyelinating and axonal. Suxamethonium is contraindicated, but the pathology of GBS is a lower motor neurone lesion. Lower motor neurone lesions treated with suxamethonium may result in dangerous potassium release.

Onset of GBS may be rapid, occurring within 48 hours. Ninety per cent of patients are maximally affected within 3–4 weeks. It generally presents with weakness spreading from the legs to the trunk and then the bulbar and facial muscles. In about 50% of cases there is a preceding respiratory or gastrointestinal illness, such as *Campylobacter* infection. Ten per cent of cases follow vaccinations. The disease is of variable duration and recovery may be complete, but damage to nerves may prolong recovery times and can leave residual weakness. Prognosis is better for the more commonly occurring demyelinating form. The axonal form may be associated with *Clostridium* infection.

Paraesthesia is common and may be a presenting symptom. Paraesthesia in GBS typically follows a glove and stocking distribution. It is one of the features that differentiate GBS from other forms of paralysis such as those associated with botulism. Tick paralysis, found in North America and Australia, is caused by neurotoxins secreted by the tick itself rather than by an infectious organism. It is similar in onset and symptoms to GBS (including para-esthesia), but recedes rapidly once the tick is removed.

Autonomic dysfunction is not uncommon and may be severe. There may be wide variations in heart rate and blood pressure, and cardiac arrest has been reported as a result of severe autonomic instability. All nerves can be affected but, in the demyelinating form, heavily myelinated nerves are affected most severely. These nerves supply motor and joint position sense (hence the weakness and paraesthesia). Pain and temperature sensation are relatively spared because the nerves supplying them are either lightly or not myelinated.

Marsh S, Pittard A. Neuromuscular disorders and anaesthesia. Part 2: specific neuromuscular disorders. *Contin Educ Anaesth Crit Care Pain* 2011; 11(4): 119–123

Rickards K, Cohen A. Guillain–Barré syndrome. *Contin Educ Anaesth Crit Care Pain* 2003; 3(2): 46–49

C8

Answer: d.

This patient is suffering from phantom limb pain. Both TENS and acupuncture have been shown to only have a short-term effect.

NSAIDs have a role only in the management of early postoperative pain not in the treatment of phantom limb pain itself. Opioids may have a role in the management of certain patients with neuropathic pain.

Mirror-box therapy has been shown to be particularly useful in the management of troublesome spasms; helping the patient to visualize the unclenching of the phantom limb.

Phantom limb pain is an intermediate indication for *spinal cord stimulation* therapy; however, stump pain responds better than phantom pain.

Jackson MA, Simpson KH. Pain after amputation. *Contin Educ Anaesth Crit Care* 2004; 4(1): 20–23

C9

Answer: b.

Nutritional requirements are often increased after brain injury and there is evidence to suggest improved outcome with the early use of enteral nutrition. It is important that electrolytes such as sodium, potassium, magnesium and phosphate are supplied with serum levels being checked. Fluid balance and serum sodium must always be carefully considered when prescribing fluids; however, a simple formula for calculating basal requirements of water is 100 ml/kg for first 10 kg, 50 ml/kg for next 10 kg and 20 ml/kg thereafter.

Calories	20–30 kcal/kg
Protein	Non-stressed patients 0.5 g/kg/day Stressed patients 1.0–1.5 g/kg/day
Glucose	2 g/kg
Na^+	1.2 mmol/kg/day
K^+	1–1.2 mmol/kg/day
Calcium	10–15 mmol/day
Phosphate	20–30 mmol/day
Fat	2 g/kg/ day

Millers RD. Chapter 95: Nutrition and metabolic control in *Miller's Anaesthesia*, Philadelphia: Churchill Livingstone, 2010

Edmonson WC. Nutritional support in critical care – an update. *Contin Educ Anaesth Crit Care Pain* 2007; 7(6): 199–202

C10

Answer: b.

The safe dose for both bupivacaine and levobupivacaine is 2 mg/kg. The child weighs 18 kg and can therefore have 36 mg bupivacaine. This equates to 7 ml of 0.5% bupivacaine or 14 mls of 0.25% bupivacaine. Adrenaline does not change the maximum safe dose of bupivacaine.

Raux O, Dadure C, Carr J, Rochette A, Capdevila X. Paediatric caudal anaesthesia. *Update Anaesth* 2010; **26**: 32–36.

C11

Answer: d.

The pain described by the patient is typical of a peripheral neuropathy (provoked, in the distribution of a nerve root and stabbing in nature). The agent of choice for management of peripheral neuropathic pain is gabapentin. Carbamazepine is cheaper but less effective, except in trigeminal neuralgia, and may cause either liver or bone marrow toxicity or both. Amitriptyline is cheaper and has similar efficacy but has more side effects and drug interactions. Duloxetine is more expensive, but is no more effective than amitriptyline.

Whilst awaiting pain clinic assessment, it is reasonable to ascend the WHO analgesic ladder.

Fine PG. Chronic pain management in older adults: special considerations. *J Pain Symp Man* 2009; **38**(2S): S4–14

C12

Answer: b.

The Brain Trauma Foundation (BTF) updated guidelines for the management of severe traumatic brain injury (TBI) describing appropriate interventions and therapeutic targets for the severely head injured patient. Intracranial pressure monitoring is recommended for all patients with severe brain injury (defined as Glasgow Coma Score 3–8) associated with an abnormal CT scan. If CT is normal, ICP monitoring is also recommended in severe head injury in the following circumstances:

- Age > 40
- Unilateral or bilateral motor posturing
- Systolic blood pressure less than 90 mmHg

There is no randomized controlled trial (RCT) evidence for improved outcomes with the use of ICP monitoring in comatose patients. However, it does allow the individualization of ICP and cerebral perfusion pressure management, whilst avoiding the detrimental consequences of treatment in patients without intracranial hypertension.

Meta-analysis of six RCTs failed to demonstrate an improvement in all-cause mortality when patients were cooled. However, an increase in the proportion of patients with good neurological outcome was suggested. The BTF suggest hypothermia as a level III recommendation only.

The recommended target for cerebral perfusion pressure in head-injured patients is 50–70 mmHg. Multiple sources have demonstrated worsened morbidity and mortality in hypotensive patients. However, aggressive maintenance of high cerebral perfusion pressure is also associated with adverse outcomes. One study, for example, demonstrated a relative risk of 5 for Acute Respiratory Distress syndrome (ARDS) when a cerebral perfusion pressure-targeted approach was compared with an ICP-targeted approach.

Aggressive hyperventilation, particularly in the first 24 hours after head injury, is not recommended because of its propensity to reduce cerebral blood flow. Multiple studies have failed to demonstrate a benefit from corticosteroids in acute head injury. Most recently the Corticosteroid Randomization After Significant Head Injury (CRASH) trial demonstrated an increased mortality in the methylprednisolone-treated cohort vs. placebo.

Brain Trauma Foundation. Guidelines for the management of severe traumatic brain injury: 3rd edn. *J. Neurotrauma* 2008; **24** (Suppl 1): S1–S106

Roberts I, Yates D, Sandercock P, *et al.* Effect of intravenous corticosteroids on death within 14 days in 10,008 adults with clinically significant head injury (MRC CRASH trial): randomised placebo controlled trial. *Lancet* 2004; **364**: 1321–1328

C13

Answer: d.

Maintenance of adequate renal perfusion pressure is essential to prevent kidney injury in these patients. This is achieved by ensuring adequate cardiac output and arterial blood pressure is maintained. Initially the patient needs aggressive intravascular fluid therapy, followed by inotropes and vasopressors if needed. Norepinephrine should be used as a first-line vasopressor as evidence does not support its adverse effects on renal, hepatic or

GI blood flow when used to maintain arterial blood pressure. Vasopressin and terlipressin are second-line drugs used in refractory cases.

Webb ST, Allen JSD. Perioperative renal protection. *Contin Educ Anaesth Crit Care Pain* 2008; 8(5): 176–180.

C14

Answer: c.

Unless there is a contraindication, it is useful to use a combination of analgesics, which will provide good pain relief with better safety profile. With an inflamed appendix and localized peritonitis, she is likely to be in quite a lot of pain postoperatively. A 3-year-old may not comprehend the use of PCA, therefore NCA is a better choice. Most general paediatric wards may not have the capacity to manage a patient on a continuous morphine infusion.

Clinical guideline: Patient controlled analgesia/nurse controlled analgesia. Great Ormond Street. http://www.gosh.nhs.uk/clinical_information/clinical_guidelines/cpg_guideline_00143/#H2_2854

C15

Answer: c.

Acute lung injury (ALI) and acute respiratory distress syndrome (ARDS) are common conditions on the ICU associated with a high mortality. ARDS is a multifactorial disease caused either by a direct insult to the lung (such as aspiration or pneumonia) or an indirect disease process (sepsis, pancreatitis, trauma). The general principles of treating ARDS are to provide optimal supportive care whilst treating the underlying cause. The only specific treatment that has been shown to significantly reduce mortality is the use of lung protective ventilation strategies. The ARDSnet group found that using low tidal volumes (6 ml/kg) and low peak inspiratory pressures (<30 cm H_2O) significantly reduced mortality. The Fluids and Catheters Treatment Trial (FACTT) compared liberal and conservative fluid management in ARDS. Conservative fluid management showed a reduction in ventilator days and ICU stay, but there was no mortality benefit. A recent meta-analysis on the use of steroids in early ARDS confirmed they confer no survival benefit. Prone positioning does improve oxygenation and reduces the incidence of ventilator-acquired pneumonia, but does not improve survival or reduce ventilator days. A systematic review of the use of inhaled nitric oxide in ALI also showed no improvement in clinical outcome.

The Acute Respiratory Distress Syndrome Network. Ventilation with lower tidal volumes as compared with traditional tidal volumes for acute lung injury and the acute respiratory distress syndrome. *N Engl J Med* 2000; **342**: 1301–1308.

Mackay A, Al-Haddad M. Acute lung injury and acute respiratory distress syndrome. *Contin Educ Anaesth Crit Care Pain* 2010; **9**(5): 152–156

C16

Answer: d.

The theoretical benefits of pre-emptive analgesia have never been translated into clinical practice. Therefore, giving diclofenac and paracetamol intra-operatively is likely to be just as effective as giving it preoperatively. Interest has shifted to 'anti-hyperalgesic' interventions using adjuvant drugs to decrease postoperative analgesic (opioid) requirements. Modification of nociceptive pathways prior to a noxious stimulus within the central nervous system by drugs such as gabapentin has been shown to have a 'protective' analgesic effect. A single preoperative dose of gabapentin has been shown to have a significant opioid-sparing effect as well as reducing anxiety levels in certain procedures. Dexamethasone has been shown to have analgesic efficacy in a number of procedures, but can be given intraoperatively. Anxious patients already taking opioids who are presenting for surgery need a thorough preoperative assessment and exploration of issues. Their usual opioid regimen should be continued perioperatively and apprehension about pain control should be allayed. Regional techniques should be considered where possible, and a multimodal analgesic approach is optimal. Anxiolytic premedication might be useful, though unlikely to directly alter analgesic requirements.

Kong VK, Irwin MG. Gabapentin: a multimodal perioperative drug? *Br J Anaesth* 2007; **99**: 775–786

C17

Answer: e.

In the UK acetaminophen overdose is the most common cause of acute hepatic failure (70%) while worldwide it is viral hepatitis. Alcohol and other drugs are implicated while *Amanita phalloides* is a poisonous mushroom and a rare cause of acute hepatic failure.

Vaja R, McNicol L, Sisley I. Anaesthesia for patients with liver disease. *Contin Educ Anaesth Crit Care Pain* 2010; **10**(1): 15–19

C18

Answer: c.

von Willebrand's disease is inherited in an autosomal dominant manner. It is the commonest inherited bleeding disorder. Typical symptoms include mucosal bleeding, easy bruising and menorrhagia. Platelet count is typically normal, the bleeding time is increased and factor VIII activity is often reduced.

von Willebrand's factor (vWF) is stored in platelets and acts as an adhesive bridge between platelets and damaged subendothelium at the site of vascular injury (primary haemostasis). It also functions as the carrier protein for factor VIII and, as such, is also involved in secondary haemostasis.

There are three main types: Type 1 (most common) has reduced amount of a functionally normal vWF. Symptoms are usually mild. Type 2 is split into four subtypes (A,B,M and N). Type 3 (least common) is the most severe form.

Datta S. (ed) Chapter 22 in *Hematologic Disease, Anaesthetic and Obstetric Management of High-Risk Pregnancy*, 3rd edn, 2004. New York: Springer

C19

Answer: b.

In the fetus most blood coming from the placenta is diverted away from the pulmonary circulation through the foramen ovale and the ductus arteriosus. At birth, pulmonary vascular resistance is lowered by lung expansion and by a reduction in hypoxic pulmonary vasoconstriction. Simultaneously, left-sided heart pressures rise by cessation of low-resistance placental flow causing an increase in systemic vascular resistance. The ductus arteriosus usually closes within 48 hours due to high PO_2 and prostaglandins.

In utero the fetal pulmonary arteries are muscular and during the early neonatal period they remain sensitive to vasoconstrictor effects of hypoxia, acidosis (hypothermia, hypercapnia) and serotonin. They are also sensitive to pulmonary vasodilators such as nitric oxide. Neonates may revert to a transitional circulation (persistent fetal circulation) if pulmonary vascular resistance increases, resulting in decrease in pulmonary blood flow and a right to left shunt through the ductus arteriosus.

In conditions such as congenital diaphragmatic hernia, respiratory distress syndrome, cardiac failure and sepsis, hypoxia and acidosis may result in pulmonary vasoconstriction, causing right to left shunting. Although the features of necrotizing enterocolitis can mimic sepsis with abdominal distension, shock and acidosis, it usually presents later (in the second week of neonatal life). The presence of ductal shunting may be demonstrated by a large difference in oxygen saturation between the arm (preductal) and the leg (postductal), with higher saturations in the arm.

Treatment consists of oxygen therapy, correction of acidosis, hypercapnia and hypothermia, inotropes and fluids. Drugs to lower pulmonary vascular resistance (e.g. isoprenaline) may be used.

Black A, McEwan A. Chapter 1: Physiology and anatomy relevant to paediatric anaesthesia, in *Paediatric and Neonatal Anaesthesia*. Michigan: Butterworth-Heinemann, 2004, 1–14

C20

Answer: d.

The advantage of the transdermal route for drug delivery is that it avoids first-pass metabolism and large variations in plasma drug concentration. Drugs must have a low molecular weight and high lipid solubility to penetrate the lipophilic stratum corneum of the skin.

There are two types of transdermal patch available: the reservoir (or membrane-controlled system) and the matrix system. In a reservoir patch the drug is held in a gel or solution and a release membrane controls the rate of delivery of the drug to the skin. The matrix patch holds the drug as part of a polymer matrix. The matrix is applied directly to the skin.

Buprenorphine and fentanyl are available as patches. They are frequently prescribed to patients with chronic non-cancer or cancer pain. The Butrans® patch is a 7-day patch delivering the opioid at 5, 10 or 20 μg per hour. This utilizes the matrix design.

Fentanyl patches are more commonly of the matrix type. The patches also deliver fentanyl at a constant rate and come in different strengths: 25 μg per hour up to 100 μg per hour. A steady-state serum concentration is achieved after 24 hours and will continue as long as the patch is renewed. Each patch lasts for 72 hours.

Because the constant delivery of drug avoids the peaks and troughs of intermittent dosaging, the side effect profile of opioids, such as sedation, nausea and vomiting and respiratory depression, is reduced. Patient compliance is also improved because of the patches' convenience.

Dose equivalence of opioid patches:

Patch	Drug delivery rate µg/h	Oral morphine mg/24 h
Butrans® 5	5	5–10
Butrans® 10	10	10–20
Butrans® 20	20	25–40
Fentanyl 12	12	20–60
Fentanyl 25	25	60–100
Fentanyl 50	50	120–200
Fentanyl 75	75	180–300
Fentanyl 100	100	240–400

Bajaj S, Whiteman A, Brander B. Transdermal drug delivery in pain management. *Cont Educ Anaesth Crit Care Pain* 2011; **11**(2): 39–43

C21

Answer: b.

St John's Wort (SJW) is widely used for the treatment of depressive disorders. Its action is thought to be due to the inhibition of the reuptake of various neurotransmitters including serotonin, dopamine and noradrenaline. In this way it has actions similar to both tricyclic antidepressants and monoamine oxidase inhibitors (MOAI). When co-administered with these medications or with some other MAOI drugs (e.g. ephedrine), as well as tyramine-containing foods, a serotoninergic syndrome can develop. This is characterized by a triad of autonomic dysfunction, altered mental function and muscle rigidity. It can also cause hyperthermic states mimicking other disorders such as malignant hyperpyrexia and neuroleptic malignant syndrome. It should be stopped before surgery if possible to minimize these interactions, but care must be taken to balance the risk of stopping antidepressant medication vs. the continuing, but with good perioperative pharmacological planning. SJW is a potent enzyme inducer, particularly of CYP2C9 (warfarin) and CYP3A4 (fentanyl/alfentayl/lignocaine/midazolam). Despite the increased metabolism of some commonly used anaesthetic medications, SJW's sedative effects can cause prolonged recovery from anaesthesia.

Wong A, Townley S. Herbal medicines and anaesthesia. *Cont Educ Anaesth Crit Care Pain* 2011; **11**(1): 14–17

C22

Answer: a.

This patient has severe pre-eclampsia (hypertension presenting after 20 weeks' gestation, with significant proteinuria, systolic blood pressure ≥ 160 mmHg and symptomatic).

Oral labetalol is the first-line treatment, aiming to keep the systolic blood pressure < 150 mmHg, and the diastolic between 80 and 100 mmHg. Caesarean section is not indicated unless the hypertension is refractory to treatment, or unless further maternal or fetal indications develop. There is no mention of eclamptic seizures prior to presentation or in a previous pregnancy; therefore magnesium sulphate is not indicated. Hydralazine and nifedipine are second-line treatments for hypertension unresponsive to labetalol.

NICE *CG107 hypertension in pregnancy: the management of hypertensive disorders during pregnancy*, 2010
NICE guidelines. Available at: http://www.nice.org.uk/nicemedia/live/13098/50418/50418. pdf (Accessed 22 February 2012)

C23

Answer: b.

The child presenting for squint surgery may be otherwise fit and well or may have associated diseases such as cerebral palsy, hydrocephalus, myopathies or other chromosomal abnormalities. Attention should be paid to these at the preoperative visit.

It is well known that strabismus surgery is associated with oculocardiac reflex. This is a bradycardic response to traction on any of the extraocular eye muscles (more commonly the medial rectus), which may also result in sinus arrest or major dysrhythmias. Afferent pathways are via the occipital branch of the trigeminal nerve and the efferent is via the vagus. Oculocardiac reflex occurs in approximately 60% of children undergoing squint surgery. On removal of traction, the bradycardia resolves almost instantaneously. Prevention will involve administering atropine 20 mcg/kg, which may be given at induction as a routine or following a reflex event in theatre.

Most cases are anaesthetized with the child spontaneously breathing, but it should be noted that light anaesthesia or hypercarbia increases the risk of oculocardiac reflex.

Strabismus surgery is associated with significant postoperative nausea and vomiting (PONV), which may be linked to oculocardiac reflex, since children who have bradycardias intraoperatively are at increased risk of PONV. Multimodal antiemetic prophylaxis should be administered.

The incidence of malignant hyperthermia is increased in patients with squint (still rare) but vigilance should be high.

James I. Anaesthesia for paediatric eye surgery. *Contin Educ Anaesth Crit Care Pain* 2008; 8(1): 5–10

C24

Answer: a.

A left-sided double lumen tube (DLT) is used most commonly for isolation of either lung. This is because there is a higher chance of occluding the right upper lobe bronchus if a right-sided tube is used.

Tidal volumes would not be halved during one-lung ventilation (OLV). Typically, 6–8 ml/kg are acceptable volumes to initiate OLV, then volumes can be titrated to limit airway pressures to an acceptable level.

Double Lumen Tube

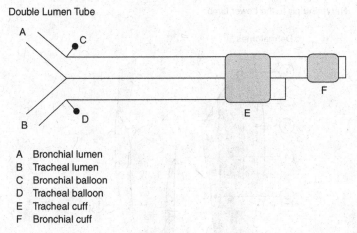

A Bronchial lumen
B Tracheal lumen
C Bronchial balloon
D Tracheal balloon
E Tracheal cuff
F Bronchial cuff

Fig. C24. Double lumen tube.

Once inserted, the DLT is connected via both lumens to the breathing circuit and both lungs are ventilated. The tracheal cuff is inflated, but the bronchial cuff will remain deflated. When OLV is required, the steps to isolate the right lung (and therefore deflate the left lung) are as follows (please refer to diagram below):

- The tracheal lumen is opened and the fresh gas flow to it is clamped (now you are ventilating only down the bronchial lumen and a leak should be heard
- Inflate the bronchial cuff until the leak disappears and you are able to auscultate breath sounds only on the left
- Unclamp the tracheal lumen (now you are ventilating both lungs)
- Open the bronchial lumen and clamp the fresh gas flow to it (this will deflate the left lung)
- Confirm there are breath sounds only on the right

The position should ideally always be confirmed with a fibre-optic bronchoscope after placement and at the time of lung isolation, particularly if the patient has been transferred or repositioned.

C25

Answer e.

This procedure requires anaesthesia of the lower leg, mostly served by the sciatic nerve. A lumbar plexus and 'three in one' do not involve the sciatic nerve, a lumbar epidural will prevent early mobilization and a posterior tibial block will only anaesthetize the foot.

Nerve Supply to the Lower Limb

Dermatomes

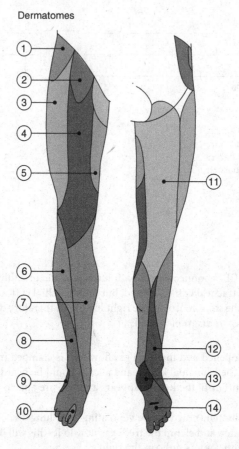

(1) Lateral cutaneous branch of subcostal nerve
(2) Femoral branch of genitofemoral nerve
(3) Lateral femoral cutaneous nerve
(4) Anterior femoral cutaneous nerves
(5) Obturator nerve
(6) Common fibular nerve
(7) Saphenous nerve
(8) Superficial fibular nerve
(9) Sural nerve
(10) Deep fibular nerve
(11) Posterior cutaneous nerve of thigh
(12) Sural nerve
(13) Calcaneal branch of tibial nerve
(14) Plantar branches of tibial nerve

Fig. C25. Nerve supply to the lower limb.

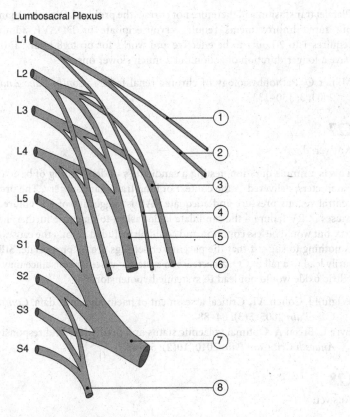

Lumbosacral Plexus

(1) Iliohypogastric nerve — L1
(2) Ilioinguinal nerve — L1
(3) Lateral femoral cutaneous nerve — L2–3
(4) Genitofemoral nerve — L1–2
(5) Femoral nerve — L2,3,4
(6) Obturator nerve — L2,3,4
(7) Sciatic nerve — L4–S2
(8) Pudendal nerve — S2,3,4

Fig. C25. (cont.)

C26

Answer: b.

Patients with CRF often bleed excessively despite normal coagulation studies. This is because of several factors causing decreased platelet adhesiveness. These are:

- Inadequate von Willebrand factor (vWF) release from the endothelium
- Increased platelet production of beta-thromboglobulin
- Increased vascular production of PGI_2
- Excessive nitric oxide

Platelet transfusion will therefore not correct the problem. Dialysis can improve the bleeding, but rapid improvements require cryoprecipitate or DDAVP administration. DDAVP requires 1 to 2 hours to be effective and works for up to 8 hours. Intravenous oestrogens have a longer duration of action but a much slower onset.

Milner Q. Pathophysiology of chronic renal failure. *Contin Educ Anaesth Crit Care Pain* 2003; **3**: 130–133

C27

Answer: d.

This is a simple question, testing a candidate's understanding of basic cardiac output study parameters; delivered in the context of lung transplant surgery. The presence of an elevated central venous pressure and adequate PAP is suggestive of RV failure. There are multiple causes of RV failure – the candidate is not asked to diagnose further; however, 'A' could be true but would be less common and could be included among the causes of RV failure. There is nothing to suggest that the pacemaker settings are inappropriate. SIRS would not necessarily lead to a fall in CO: a decrease in systemic vascular resistance may in fact increase CO. Nitric oxide would not lead to systemic hypotension.

Wigfull J, Cohen AT. Critical assessment of haemodynamic data. *Contin Educ Anaesth Crit Care Pain* 2005; **5**(3): 84–88
Eyre L, Breen A. Optimal volaemic status and predicting fluid responsiveness. *Contin Educ Anaesth Crit Care Pain* 2010; **10**(2): 59–62

C28

Answer: d.

Recommendations from the consensus group of the American Society of Regional Anaesthesia are that needle placement in patients receiving prophylactic doses of LMWH should be 10–12 hours after the previous dose of LMWH. In those receiving higher therapeutic doses, placement should be delayed at least 24 hours. The APTT ratio is used to monitor the administration of unfractionated heparin and the PT ratio to monitor warfarin administration. Neither are appropriate tests to monitor LMWH administration. An anti factor 10a assay is available; however, it has not been shown to be predictive of the risk of bleeding.

Regional anesthesia in the patient receiving antithrombotic or thrombolytic therapy. American Society of Regional Anesthesia and Pain Medicine Evidence-Based Guidelines, 3rd edn. *Regional Anesth Pain Med* 2010; **35**(1): 64–101

C29

Answer: d.

'Muscular dystrophy' is a group of congenital conditions, characterized by progressive muscle weakness. Boys are more commonly affected than girls. There are several subtypes of muscular dystrophy, including Duchenne's, Becker's and Emery–Dreifuss. Pathologically, the disease affects skeletal, cardiac and smooth muscle.

Implications for anaesthesia:

- Risk of aspiration due to decreased gut motility, delayed gastric emptying and dysphagia. Consider preoperative antacid premedication.
- Reduced doses of non-depolarizing neuromuscular blockers should be used due to increased sensitivity.
- Postoperative respiratory insufficiency. Consider preoperative lung function tests.
- Pre-existing cardiomyopathy; myocardial dysfunction can be significantly exacerbated by myocardial depressant anaesthetic drugs.
- Suxamethonium-induced hyperkalaemia and rhabdomyolysis. This reaction can be potentially fatal, and is known to be associated with several forms of muscular dystrophy. It appears to resemble malignant hyperthermia; volatile agents may also be a trigger. However, a concurrent rise in temperature is not always seen. The current consensus is that malignant hyperthermia triggers should be avoided in muscular dystrophy patients. Thus, propofol TIVA is the most appropriate technique.

Allman KG, Wilson IH (ed). *Oxford Handbook of Anaesthesia, 3rd edn*. 2011. Oxford: Oxford University Press

Hayes J, Veykemans F, Bissonnette B. Duchenne muscular dystropy: an old anaesthesia problem revisited. *Paediatr Anaesth* 2008; **18**: 100–106

C30

Answer: c.

Obstructive sleep apnoea is associated with frequent periods of hypoventilation and/or apnoeas during sleep, with resultant episodic hypoxaemia. Diagnosis is based upon a supportive history of loud snoring, perhaps with witnessed apnoeas, and daytime somnolence as well as evidence of risk factors such as obesity, enlarged tonsils/adenoids, craniofacial abnormalities or neuromuscular disorders. Objective testing can be as simple as watching a patient sleep whilst measuring their oxygen saturations. The 'gold standard' is more expensive and time consuming – polysomnography. This involves the measurement of several physiological parameters during sleep. Electroencephalogram (EEG), electromyogram (EMG) and electro-oculogram (EOG) information is recorded whilst the patient passes through the four stages of sleep with REM and non-REM sleep being easily differentiated. Air flow is measured by the use of a flow sensor or thermistor mounted near the patient's nose. Oxygen saturations are recorded via a saturations monitor. Sometimes measurements of respiratory effort are recorded from an oesophageal pressure sensor or inferred from diaphragmatic EMG recordings. Other information such as ECG and blood pressure may also be noted. The data are then analysed in 30-second segments and information is obtained on the frequency and magnitude of desaturations, and the cardiovascular variations associated with arousal episodes. End-tidal carbon dioxide measurements are not normally recorded.

Martinez G, Faber P. Obstructive sleep apnoea. *Contin Educ Anaesth Crit Care Pain* 2011; **11**(1): 5–8

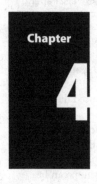

Questions – Paper D

D1

A 56-year-old man with severe claustrophobia requires a general anaesthetic for an MRI scan of his entire spine.

Regarding monitoring in the MRI scanner, which of the following would be the most appropriate combination of patient monitors in addition to a fibre-optic pulse oximeter?
a. Three ECG electrodes placed in the CM5 position and a non-invasive blood pressure cuff (NIBP)
b. Four ECG electrodes placed less than 20 cm apart, a NIBP cuff
c. Four ECG electrodes placed more than 20 cm apart, an arterial line
d. Three ECG electrodes placed less than 20 cm apart, a NIBP cuff
e. Three ECG electrodes placed less than 20 cm apart, an arterial line

D2

Total intravenous anaesthesia (TIVA) is a commonly used anaesthetic technique. A number of pharmacokinetic models exist which may be used to control drug delivery.

Which of the following is the most accurate statement?
a. The Marsh model for propofol would result in the delivery of a lower total propofol dose than the Schneider model in the same patient if used at the same target concentrations
b. The Marsh model is suitable for use in morbidly obese patients
c. Using the Marsh model in paediatric patients is more likely to result in awareness than in adults
d. The Minto model for remifentanil uses actual body weight in its calculations
e. TIVA should not be used in children because of the risk of propofol infusion syndrome

D3

A 54-year-old man presents for a sigmoid colectomy for a colonic cancer. He is taking warfarin for a deep venous thrombosis that occurred 3 months previously. His warfarin will be stopped 5 days preoperatively and his INR checked on the evening before surgery.

While the warfarin is stopped, the following should be commenced:
a. Aspirin 150 mg daily.
b. Intravenous unfractionated heparin titrated to a PTT of 2.5 times greater than control.

Practice Single Best Answer Questions for the Final FRCA, ed. Hozefa Ebrahim, Khalid Hasan, Mark Tindall, Michael Clarke and Natish Bindal. Published by Cambridge University Press. © Cambridge University Press 2013.

c. Enoxaparin 0.5 mg/kg daily
d. Aspirin 75 mg and clopidogrel 75 mg daily
e. Enoxaparin 0.5 mg/kg 12-hourly

D4

A 30-year-old male is undergoing general anaesthesia for appendicectomy. He has had a previous anaphylactic reaction to suxamethonium. You have performed a rapid sequence induction with rocuronium 1.2 mg/kg. You are unable to intubate or ventilate. A laryngeal mask airway is *in situ*, but you remain unable to ventilate the patient. He is cyanosed and bradycardic.

What do you do next?
a. Give Suggamadex 16 mg kg^{-1} and administer high-flow oxygen via facemask
b. Re-attempt intubation with a McCoy's blade
c. Give 100% oxygen and call for senior assistance
d. Oxygenate via needle cricothyroidotomy
e. Administer 600 mcg atropine

D5

Healthcare-associated infections (HCAIs) are a significant burden to health services. The anaesthetist plays a pivotal role in the prevention of transmission of such infections. One area of responsibility is to ensure that all anaesthetic equipment is effectively decontaminated.

Regarding the decontamination of anaesthetic equipment, which of the following is correct?
a. Fibre-optic endoscopes are autoclaved at 134 °C
b. Prions should all be removed after five decontamination cycles
c. Laryngoscope handles should be sterilized after every patient, or disposable handles used
d. Chemical indicators are used in sterile packs to confirm that the contents are sterile
e. A 70% alcohol and chlorhexidine mixture is a high-level disinfectant

D6

A 28-year-old female presents to the emergency department following a drug overdose. She is known to mental health services. Shortly after arrival, she develops vomiting, abdominal pain and lethargy. She later complains of severe blurred vision and is noted to have a severe muscle twitching. An hour later she has a grand mal seizure.

The most likely drug is:
a. Codeine phosphate
b. Diazepam
c. Paracetamol
d. Amitriptyline
e. Lithium

D7

Combined spinal–epidural (CSE) anaesthesia aims to provide rapid relief and a long duration of action. There are a number of techniques and a wide variety of situations in which this technique may be useful.

Which of the following is most accurate?
a. The paramedian approach is not suitable for CSE
b. The Royal College of Anaesthetists 'NAP3' audit shows that around 6% of neuraxial blocks are CSEs
c. An epidural top up should be injected immediately after the spinal injection is given
d. CSEs are associated with a four-fold increase in PDPH
e. Proportionally fewer CSEs result in major harm than either epidurals or spinals performed alone

D8

A 40-year-old female presents for a trans-sphenoidal resection of a pituitary tumour.

Which of the following does not indicate an excess of growth hormone secretion?
a. Retrognathism
b. Macroglossia
c. Obstructive sleep apnoea
d. Cardiomyopathy
e. Impaired glucose tolerance

D9

A 45-year-old woman attends the chronic pain clinic; she has had spontaneous widespread pain for 4 months. Her history and examination reveal a widespread pain index (WP) value of 9. She is suffering from altered sleep and fatigue. She is diagnosed with fibromyalgia based upon the American College of Rheumatologists (ACR) criteria.

Which of the following is the most appropriate first-line treatment?
a. Amitriptyline 10 mg at night
b. Fluoxetine 20 mg daily
c. Injection of identified trigger points with local anaesthetic and corticosteroid
d. Tramadol 50–100 mg four times daily
e. Gabapentin at a starting dose of 300 mg, increasing daily

D10

A 53-year-old male was admitted to the intensive care unit 4 days previously with severe traumatic brain injury after a road traffic collision. He remains comatose despite cessation of sedation.

Which of the following would be the most appropriate method for exclusion of significant cervical spine injury in this patient?
a. A combination of plain-film cervical radiography and dynamic fluoroscopy
b. Dynamic cervical fluoroscopy alone
c. Cervical magnetic resonance imaging (MRI)
d. A combination of plain-film cervical radiography and helical computed tomography (CT)
e. Plain-film cervical radiography alone

D11

You attend a trauma call where a 34-year-old male has been involved in a road traffic collision. He was intubated on scene due to a GCS of 6 and has a single 20G cannula in the left hand. The primary survey reveals markedly reduced breath sounds on the right side of the chest, pulse of 110 bpm and a blood pressure of 70/ 30 mmHg. He has bruising over the right flank.

Which of the following is the next most appropriate step in his management?
a. Right side needle thoracocentesis
b. Right side tube thoracostomy
c. Establish large bore access and commence volume replacement
d. Open thoracotomy
e. Ultrasound scan to rule out intra-abdominal bleed

D12

An 8-kg 11-month-old child is undergoing a circumcision. The anaesthetist decides to perform a caudal anaesthetic.

What volume of 0.25% bupivacaine is required to achieve a lumbosacral blockade in this child?
a. 2 ml
b. 4 ml
c. 6 ml
d. 8 ml
e. 10 ml

D13

A GP has referred a 56-year-old lady who is 6 months post fracture of the ankle and complains of ongoing ankle and foot pain that is not responsive to simple analgesics. Repeat ankle X-ray shows no significant abnormality.

In the management of complex regional pain syndrome (CRPS):
a. CRPS type 2 is often initiated by peripheral nerve transection
b. Topical NSAIDs are more effective than systemic preparations
c. CRPS type 1 generally follows major trauma to major nerves and is characterized by diffuse pain distal to the injury
d. If sympathetic blocks are successful, then neurolysis is the treatment of choice in most cases
e. Vasomotor instability is a feature of CRPS types 1 and 2

D14

Community-acquired pneumonias are commonly seen and may be severe, requiring anaesthetic or ICU input. Knowledge of the causative agents and first-line treatments can improve outcomes.

Concerning community-acquired pneumonias, which statement is most accurate?
a. Streptococci commonly produce β-lactamases
b. Legionellae are Gram-positive organisms
c. Staphylococci are generally coagulase negative
d. *Chlamydia pneumoniae* is generally insensitive to fluoroquinolones
e. *Coxiella burnetti* is β-lactam sensitive

D15

You are asked to review an 82-year-old man on ICU following an emergency aortic aneurysm repair 5 days ago. Despite his observations being stable throughout the day, he has become increasingly confused and appears to be having visual hallucinations. He has pulled out his nasogastric tube and arterial line and is trying to get out of bed, despite reassurance.

What would be the best initial treatment?
a. 2.5 mg intravenous haloperidol
b. Oxygen via a non-rebreathe mask
c. 4 mg intravenous lorazepam
d. Application of physical restraints to prevent injury to himself or others
e. Melatonin and dexmedetomidine

D16

You have been asked to anaesthetize an ex-premature baby, born at 32 weeks' gestation, for elective bilateral inguinal hernia repair. His corrected gestational age is 60 weeks and he weighs 3.5 kg. He was discharged home 24 weeks ago without ancillary oxygen and has been well in himself.

What would be your preferred anaesthetic technique?
a. Caudal block with sedation
b. General anaesthesia with 0.3 mg of intravenous morphine and intravenous infusion of paracetamol 22.5 mg
c. General anaesthesia with bilateral ilioinguinal blocks
d. General anaesthesia with caudal block
e. Spinal anaesthesia with sedation

D17

A 20-year-old female with Ehlers–Danlos syndrome has long-term pain due to recurrent hip dislocations. She is using and seeking increasing doses of oral morphine solution to manage this. Despite this, her pain is poorly controlled and it is later discovered that she has not been able to re-locate her hip for some time.

What term best describes her behaviour?
a. Addiction
b. Pseudo-addiction
c. Tolerance
d. Physical dependence
e. Craving

D18

Recipients of solid organ transplants may require other surgery.

The priorities in preoperative assessment are:
a. Liaising with the organ transplantation team to see when the patient was last reviewed
b. Limiting the amount of perioperative fluids to avoid dilution of the serum levels of immunosuppressive drugs

c. Avoiding drugs that are metabolized by the cytochrome P-450 enzyme pathway, as they may interfere with cyclosporine or tacrolimus levels
d. Using a regional anaesthetic technique if possible
e. Assessment of the function of the graft and detecting the complications associated with immunosuppressive therapy

D19

You have been asked to provide an epidural for a labouring mother. Your patient is a lawyer specializing in medical negligence. She wishes to know in detail about the risks of an epidural.

Which of the following statements is incorrect?
a. The risk of a postdural puncture headache is about 1 in 100
b. The risk of a temporary nerve injury is about 1 in 1000
c. The risk of a meningitis is about 1 in 100 000
d. The risk of not working well enough so that alternative analgesia is required is about 1 in 8
e. The risk of needing an instrumental delivery is about 1 in 15

D20

A 10-year-old boy has fallen out of a tree and broken his arm. He is listed for open reduction and internal fixation on your trauma list. He is third on your list and the first two cases are likely to take 2 hours. He is complaining of pain in his arm, which he scores as 6 out of 10 on a visual analogue scale and, other than receiving a 15-mg/kg dose of oral paracetamol on admission (1 hour ago), he has not received any other analgesia.

What would be the most appropriate pharmacological management of his pain?
a. Rectal diclofenac 1 mg/kg and oral codeine 1 mg/kg
b. Additional 15 mg/kg of oral paracetamol
c. Intravenous morphine bolus 0.1 mg/kg
d. Oral ibuprofen 5 mg/kg and codeine 1 mg/kg
e. Inhaled entonox

D21

You are assessing a 39-year-old male in your chronic pain management clinic. He gives you a 6-month history of pain in his lower back. There is no history of trauma and he is otherwise well. Your examination is unremarkable. He takes regular paracetamol and ibuprofen, which slightly ease the pain.

After discussing analgesic options, what would be the next step in your management of this patient?
a. Offer a course of physical therapy
b. Offer transcutaneous electrical nerve stimulation (TENS)
c. Prescribe gabapentin
d. Request a lumbar spine MRI
e. Request a lumbar spine X-ray

D22

Clinical tests may be used to prove or disprove the occurrence of a disease, or to guide its management. These tests should accurately spot all patients who have the disease and also all those who are free from it.

Which of the following statements regarding clinical tests is true?
a. A clinical test is 100% sensitive if it identifies all patients without the disease
b. A clinical test is 100% specific if it identifies all patients with the disease
c. The positive predictive value (PPV) of a test determines the likelihood of a patient not having the disease if they test positive for it
d. The negative predictive value (NPV) of a test determines the probability of actually correctly diagnosing people without disease if they test negative
e. The likelihood ratio of a clinical test predicts the odds of having the disease when the test is negative

D23

A 36-year-old patient presents in labour to your district general hospital. She has known rheumatic aortic stenosis with a mean valvular gradient of 55 mmHg. On examination by the midwife, she is found to have cervical dilatation of 6 cm. She is now asking for pain relief. You have sited an arterial line for close blood pressure monitoring and transferred her to the obstetric HDU room.

Which of the following best describes an appropriate plan for her intra-partum management?
a. Combined spinal–epidural for analgesia and aim for vaginal delivery
b. Early, semi-elective Caesarean under GA
c. Epidural for analgesia, and consideration of instrumental delivery early during the second stage
d. Epidural for analgesia, with a plan to use 'quick-mix' solution (1 ml 8.4% bicarbonate, 0.1 ml '1 in1000' epinephrine, made up to 20 ml with 2% lidocaine) to achieve appropriate anaesthesia for operative delivery if required
E. Pulmonary artery catheterization, fluid resuscitation titrated to a pulmonary artery wedge pressure of 5–12 mmHg, epidural for analgesia and allow the patient to labour normally

D24

A 7-year-old girl presents to the emergency department following a suspected accidental drug overdose whilst playing in a garage. She is confused with slurred speech, mydriasis and an ataxic gait. Later, she complains of nausea and is tachypnoeic. A venous blood gas shows a severe metabolic acidosis and a BM of 7 mmol/l. After 1 hour she has a generalized tonic–clonic seizure.

What is the most likely drug that has been ingested?
a. Ethylene glycol
b. Tramadol
c. Aspirin
d. Organophosphates
e. Amitriptyline

D25

When a patient undergoes deep hypothermic circulatory arrest (DHCA) during aortic arch repair, all the following are consequences except:

a. Left-shift in the oxygen dissociation curve
b. Decreased cerebral metabolic rate by a factor of 2.6 for every 10-degree drop in temperature
c. Extracellular alkalosis
d. Altered rheology
e. Cerebral blood flow (CBF) autoregulation maintained with pH-stat blood gas management

D26

A 78-year-old female is undergoing an emergency uncemented hemi-arthroplasty under general anaesthesia with associated lumbar plexus block. Following the insertion of the prosthesis into the femoral shaft, the surgeon relocates the prosthesis into the joint. Within 2 minutes the end-tidal CO_2 falls from 4.6 kPa to 1.2 kPa, the pulse rate remains between 70 and 80 bpm and the blood pressure recorded is 50 mmHg systolic.

What is the most likely cause?
a. Bone-cement-induced hypotension
b. Endotracheal tube displacement
c. Local anaesthetic toxicity
d. Massive fat embolism
e. Acute hypovolaemia

D27

You are due to anaesthetize a 32-year-old male who is normally anuric with end-stage renal disease for his renal transplant. He has no other cardiorespiratory comorbidities and was last dialysed 24 hours previously.

As part of your preoperative assessment you would most importantly confirm he has:
a. No history of recent infection
b. Received intravenous fluids for the period of starvation
c. Been given ranitidine
d. Had platelet function tests
e. Had a potassium check at least within 6 hours of induction

D28

Pharmacokinetics of anaesthetic drugs in the morbidly obese patient changes significantly. Which of the following statements with regard to anaesthetic drug dosing in the morbidly obese is true?

a. Thiopentone sodium dose for induction is calculated according to total body weight
b. The dose of suxamethonium is calculated on the basis of lean body weight ·
c. The dose of hyperbaric bupivacaine 0.5% for subarachnoid block should be halved
d. Rocuronium dose depends on total body weight
e. Propofol used as infusion for total intravenous anaesthesia (TIVA) should be based upon total body weight

D29

You assess a 65-year-old gentleman scheduled for an elective abdominal aortic aneurysm repair the following day. You notice he is not currently taking beta-blockers.

Regarding the initiation of therapy, which of the following is appropriate?
a. 50 mg metoprolol orally 2 hours preoperatively
b. 5 mg atenolol intravenously prior to induction, titrated to heart rate
c. Postpone and give 2.5 mg bisoprolol for three days prior to surgery
d. Postpone and give 2.5 mg bisoprolol initially, for at least a week prior to surgery, dose titrated to heart rate
e. Beta-blockers are not indicated in this case

D30

You are asked to anaesthetize a 30-year-old male for resection of an abdominal phaeochromocytoma.

Your preoperative assessment should focus on:
a. Detecting a high haematocrit, as it is a reliable indicator of volaemic status
b. Searching for associations, such as in multiple endocrine neoplasia (MEN) 2A.
c. Assessment of the sympathetic blockade by α and β antagonists, with an adequately controlled heart rate and blood pressure.
d. Achieving good premedication with temazepam
e. Arranging an intensive care or high dependency bed postoperatively.

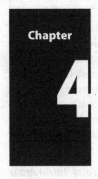

Chapter

4

Paper D – Answers

D1

Answer: b.

Monitoring in the MRI scanner presents a number of challenges. Interference with the biological signal is the main problem, as the powerful magnetic field induces electrical current in wires such as ECG leads and the pulse oximeter. To minimize this, the optimum configuration of ECG leads is to use four leads placed less than 20 cm apart in a square formation in the centre of the chest. The leads are attached to non-ferromagnetic electrodes and have braided shielded wires to dissipate any induced currents to earth. ST analysis is not reliable.

The pulse oximeter has standard red and infra LEDs at the patient end, but the signal is transmitted to the monitor via a fibre-optic cable to minimize interference. These are fragile and expensive to replace if damaged.

The majority of arterial line transducers are compatible in the MRI scanner, but there are usually few problems with NIBP monitoring using compatible cuffs.

The other consideration regarding monitoring is the heating effect produced by induced electrical currents in monitoring leads. To minimize the risk of thermal injury to the patient, the leads should never be in direct contact with the skin and coiling of the leads should be avoided.

Osborn I. Magnetic resonance imaging anesthesia. *Curr Opin Anesthesiol* 2002; **15**: 443–448

D2

Answer: c.

The Marsh and Schneider models are very different and result in a dissimilar pattern of drug delivery. The Schneider model usually delivers a smaller loading dose and total dose than the Marsh would in the same patient. It is important to receive adequate training and have a sufficient knowledge of the model before it is used in clinical practice.

The Marsh model has been shown to under-dose children under the age of 16 and therefore its use should be restricted to adults. Care must be taken in obese patients as the model will attempt to calculate lean body weight from the inputted value, which may actually become negative if the value is too high due to the formula used for the calculation. The Minto model for remifentanil uses lean body mass, but actual weight can be inputted into the device.

Propofol-related infusion syndrome (PRIS) is a rare but life-threatening condition seen more commonly in children and critically ill patients who have received prolonged infusions of propofol, usually in a dose exceeding 4 mg/kg per hour for greater than 48 hours. There have been isolated case reports of PRIS during prolonged anaesthesia, but there is insufficient evidence to suggest that TIVA is contra-indicated in children. However, it is generally not used to sedate children on intensive care. The syndrome is characterized by rhabdomyolysis (of skeletal and cardiac muscle) and the rapid development of a metabolic acidosis and multiorgan dysfunction.

Absalom A, Struys M. *Overview of Target Controlled Infusions and Total Intravenous Anaesthesia*. Academia Press, 2005.

Fordale V, LA Monaca E. Propofol infusion syndrome: an overview of a perplexing disease. *Drug Saf Update* 2008; **31**(4):293–303

D3

Answer: e.

This patient has had a provoked DVT. The provocation, colonic malignancy, has not resolved and he is less than 6 months from the occurrence of the DVT, placing him at high risk of perioperative recurrence. He thus qualifies for extended rather than for standard prophylaxis. Neither aspirin nor clopidogrel is effective in this setting. Intravenous unfractionated heparin will require admission and carries the risk of causing heparin-induced thrombocytopaenia (HIT).

Douketis JD (2009). Perioperative management of antithrombotic therapy: lifting the fog. *J Thromb Haemost*; 7: 1979–1981

D4

Answer: d.

There are a number of generic core airway skills required of an anaesthetist and described in the documentation of the Royal College of Anaesthetists. This question tests knowledge of the 'can't intubate, can't ventilate' scenario with increasing hypoxaemia.

This is an airway emergency in a patient who is about to suffer a hypoxaemic cardiac arrest. The treatment of this periarrest situation is to reverse the hypoxaemic state. Attempts to manage the airway so far have failed and there is no place for further attempts at intubation or for using a fibre-optic scope to site an endotracheal tube.

The answer is to perform a rescue airway technique to treat hypoxaemia. Options include surgical or needle cricothyroidotomy. As surgical cricothyroidotomy is not given as an option, the answer must be needle cricothyroidotomy. Atropine, although a treatment for bradycardia is not the treatment of choice in this setting as treatment of hypoxaemia is paramount.

Sugammadex, used for reversal of neuromuscular blockade by rocuronium could be given but in this setting will take several minutes to reverse the effects if given at a dose of 16 mg/kg. This therefore would not be your first action at this stage. Priority is to oxygenate the patient.

Difficult Airway Society guidelines flowchart 2004 is available at www.das.uk.com

D5

Answer: c.

Decontamination is the term used to describe a combination of processes used to make a reusable item safe to handle by staff and safe for further patient use. It includes cleaning, disinfection and/or sterilization.

Cleaning is the physical removal of foreign material and may not destroy infective organisms at all. It is, however, very important for the removal of spores.

Disinfection is a process that eliminates many or all pathogenic organisms. Low-level disinfection kills most vegetative bacteria but not all fungi, viruses or endospores. Seventy per cent alcohol with chlorhexidine is a low-level disinfectant. High-level disinfectants such as peracetic acid kill most organisms.

Sterilization is a process used to render an object free from all viable micro-organisms including bacteria, viruses and spores. Autoclaving, glutaraldehyde and ethylene oxide are all methods of sterilization.

Prions can be transmitted from certain tissues in the body such as the tonsils, lymph tissue, appendix and brain tissue. They can survive up to ten cycles of decontamination. The diseases transmitted can be spongiform encephalopathies such as variant Creutzfeldt–Jakob disease (vCJD).

Fibre-optic scopes cannot be autoclaved; they are disinfected in an automated washer.

Chemical indicators are used on sterile packs, but will only indicate that the appropriate processes have been followed; they are no guarantee of sterility.

It is recommended that all laryngoscope blades and handles are either decontaminated between patients or fully disposable laryngoscopes are deployed. There have been reports of infections being passed on from laryngoscope handles, therefore it is important to change the handles as well as the blades.

AAGBI guideline – *Infection Control in Anaesthesia*. Revised 2008.

D6

Answer: e.

When one considers the previous psychiatric history and the constellation of signs and symptoms, the most likely drug is lithium. This is thought to be due to lithium mimicking the physiological effects of sodium. For anaesthesia, it is highly relevant as lithium prolongs both depolarizing and non-depolarizing muscle relaxants. Generalized seizures are rare in opioid toxicity, though commoner in children due to the initial CNS excitation. The effects of amitriptyline toxicity are tachycardia, hypotension, impaired myocardial contractility, arrhythmias (VT, VF) and coma, among other muscarinic effects.

Flood S, Bodenham A. Lithium: mimicry, mania, and muscle relaxants. *Contin Educ Anaesth Crit Care Pain* 2010; **10**(3): 77–80.

D7

Answer: b.

There are a number of methods of performing a CSE, but none have been shown to be superior. Studies so far are limited, but show that any of the available methods are effective by either the paramedian or midline approaches and that there is no additional risk of any of the associated ill effects.

The Royal College of Anaesthetists Third National Audit Project gives details of neuraxial blocks performed over a year between 1 September 2006 and 31 August 2007. It gives details of the number of cases of neuraxial block-related haematoma, infection, paralysis and a range of other complications. The results of the audit show that around 6% of neuraxial blocks performed in that year were in CSEs and that these led to around 15% of the major complications. The Royal College Audits are mandatory reading for all anaesthetists, particularly those intending to pass their FRCA.

Cook TM, Counsell D, Wildsmith JAW on behalf of The Royal College of Anaesthetists Third National Audit Project. (2009) Major complications of central neuraxial block: report on the Third National Audit Project of the Royal College of Anaesthetists. *Br J Anaesth* 2009; **102** *(2)*: 179–190

Ong Kar-Binh, Sashidharan R. Combined spinal–epidural techniques. *Contin Educ Anaesth Crit Care Pain* 2007; **7**(2): 38–41

D8

Answer: a.

All of the above except retrognathism are features of acromegaly as a result of a pituitary adenoma. Retrognathism (receding jaw) is not associated with growth hormone (GH) excess, as the condition is more associated with continued growth of the facial bones and this tends to result in mandibular protrusion.

Excessive GH in the adult stimulates production of IGF-1 and this tends to result in excessive growth of soft tissue, cartilage and bones in the face, hands and feet. Other features include:
- hypertrophy of soft tissues, viscera, and skin. This leads to mucosal polyps, skin tags, thickened skin and carpal tunnel syndrome
- excessive soft tissue growth of the upper airways can lead to obstructive sleep apnoea, hoarseness (recurrent laryngeal nerve palsy) and laryngeal narrowing. Macrognathia, macroglossia and increased distance between incisors are also features
- hirsutism
- cardiomyopathy, hypertension, ischaemic heart disease and valvular disorders
- diabetes – hyperglycaemia may be as a direct result of GH secretion but diabetes is more common in patients with acromegaly. Pre-existing diabetes may become more difficult to control
- proximal myopathy, arthritis
- tumours – uncontrolled GH levels are associated with increased risk of tumours, including colonic polyps and uterine fibroids
- reduced life expectancy – this can be reduced by approximately 10 years, if GH levels are uncontrolled and in the presence of diabetes and heart disease

Surgery is generally via a trans-sphenoidal approach, performed through the nose or by an incision under the upper lip. Preoperative assessment should pay particular attention to airway involvement and the other effects of GH excess outlined above (especially diabetes and cardiovascular disease). One should also be aware of other hormone deficiency, e.g.

hypoadrenalism (hyponatraemia, hypovolaemia) or hypothyroidism, and supplement accordingly.

Menon R, Murphy PG, Lindley AM. Anaesthesia and pituitary disease. *Contin Educ Anaesth Crit Care Pain* 2011; **11**(4): 133–137

D9

Answer: a.

Fibromyalgia is diagnosed based on criteria laid down by the ACR. Firstly, widespread spontaneous chronic pain for a period of greater than 3 months; the extent of pain is then assessed using the widespread pain index (WPI) and other symptoms are assessed using a symptom severity (SS) scale. Criteria for the diagnosis of fibromyalgia include a WPI>7 and SS>5 or WPI 3–6 and SS>9.

Pharmacological treatment of choice is amitriptyline, a tricyclic antidepressant (TCA), it has actions including inhibition of reuptake of 5-HT and norepinephrine. TCAs may also help with other symptoms including improving quality of sleep. SSRIs such as fluoxetine may improve mood and fatigue but have little effect on pain. Weak opioids have been used, but their use is limited by side effects.

Trigger point injections may be used but are not a first-line treatment.

Dedhia JD, Bone ME. Pain and fibromyalgia. *Contin Educ Anaesth Crit Care Pain* 2009; **9**(5): 162–166

Wolfe F, Clauw DJ, Fitzcharles MA *et al.* The American College of Rheumatology Preliminary Diagnostic Criteria for Fibromyalgia and Measurement of Symptom Severity. *Arthritis Care Res* 2010; **62**: 600–610

D10

Answer: d.

Approximately one-third of head injuries are associated with cervical spine injury. Moreover, the presence of a significant head injury may impair the clinician's ability to assess the patient's cervical spine. Prolonged spinal immobilization is associated with a number of complications including skin ulceration, thromboembolism, gastrointestinal dysfunction and hospital-acquired infections. It is therefore desirable to apply a pragmatic approach for 'clearing' the cervical spine in patients in whom clinical examination is impossible, and in whom the risks of prolonged immobilization are likely to outweigh the benefits.

Numerous imaging modalities have been suggested as appropriate in such circumstances, including computed tomography (CT), magnetic resonance imaging (MRI) and dynamic cervical fluoroscopy. There is limited evidence that any of these techniques are superior. Plain-film radiography alone is certainly insufficient, since up to 15% of injuries may remain undiagnosed. Approximately 0.1%–1% of cervical spine injuries are missed by a combination of cervical radiography and CT. The sensitivity of this technique is therefore comparable to dynamic fluoroscopy and MRI.

The Intensive Care Society published guidelines in 2005 suggesting that unconscious polytrauma patients should undergo clearing of the cervical spine within 48 to 72 hours of injury. Lateral and AP radiographs, together with helical CT scanning from the cranio-cervical junction to C7 were suggested as sufficient. The routine use of dynamic fluoroscopy or MRI were not recommended.

Morris CG, McCoy EP, Lavery GG. Spinal immobilisation for unconscious patients with multiple injuries. *Br Med J* 2004; **329**: 495–499

D11

Answer: c.

The most likely diagnosis is a right-sided haemothorax and requires a relatively large chest drain to be inserted urgently. A considerable amount of blood can accumulate in the pleural space and it is important to establish large-bore intravenous access and have fluids ready to commence prior to insertion of the chest drain. According to ATLS guidelines, emergency open thorocotomy is indicated in the event of:
- the evacuation of more than 1000 ml of blood immediately after tube thoracostomy
- continued bleeding from the chest – defined as 150–200 ml/h for 2–4 hours
- repeated blood transfusion is required to maintain hemodynamic stability

American College of Surgeons Committee on Trauma. *Advanced Trauma Life Support (ATLS) for Doctors; Student Course Manual*, 8th edn, 2008. Chicago: American College of Surgeons.

D12

Answer: b.

The Armitage formula, which uses 0.25% bupivacaine or 0.2% ropivacaine states that, for a lumbosacral block, 0.5 ml/kg is required. For a thoracolumbar block, 1 ml/kg and for a mid-thoracic 1.25 ml/kg is required.

Raux O, Dadure C, Carr J, Rochette A, Capdevila X. Paediatric caudal anaesthesia. *Update Anaesth* 2010; **26**: 32–36

D13

Answer: e.

CRPS type 1 is characterized by diffuse pain following damage to structures not including nerves. CRPS type 2 is generally associated with nerve damage but not transection and is characterized by pain in the distribution of the affected nerve.

Topical preparations are often ineffective, although capsaicin may be useful in some cases.

Neurolysis is not necessarily the next step after sympathetic blocks. The blocks are often repeated and can either increase or decrease in efficacy.

Vasomotor instability is a common feature of both subtypes of CRPS. They are similar in many respects, the major differences being in their causes and the distribution of the pain which results.

Pickering A. An overview of neuropathic pain. *Contin Educ Anaesth Crit Care Pain* 2002; **2** (3): 65–68

Wilson J, Serpell M. Complex regional pain syndrome. *Contin Educ Anaesth Crit Care Pain* 2007; 7(2): 51–54

D14

Answer: c.

β-Lactamase-producing streptococci are uncommon in the UK and resistance to penicillins appears to be decreasing. Staphylococci are generally coagulase negative, but *Staphylococcus aureus* is different in that it is coagulase positive. The atypicals, which include *Mycoplasma pneumoniae, Chlamydia pneumoniae, Chlamydia psittaci* and *Coxiella burnetii* are generally insensitive to penicillins and require treatment with other antibiotics. Macrolides, tetracyclines and fluoroquinolones can be used depending on specific types.

Sadashivaiah JB, Carr B. Severe community-acquired pneumonia. *Contin Educ Anaesth Crit Care Pain* 2009; 9(3): 87–91

D15

Answer: a.

Delirium in critically ill patients is a common occurrence. Delirium is associated with increased mortality, infection rates and increased length of hospital stay. The cause is usually multi-factorial. Risk factors for delirium include: old age, alcoholism, smoking, visual/ hearing impairment, sepsis/pyrexia, sleep disturbance, immobilization and medication.

Hyperactive delirium occurs in 5%–22% of patients. The majority of critically ill patients with delirium have either the hypoactive form or a mixed picture, where they fluctuate between having hyperactive and hypoactive states. Hypoactive delirium is commonly missed.

A multi-modal approach to management is most likely to be effective. Risk factors should be addressed. If simple methods fail, then pharmacological treatment may be required. The Society of Critical Care Medicine and the American Psychiatric Association recommend haloperidol as the first-line drug of choice, or olanzapine if haloperidol is not tolerated. Benzodiazepines should be avoided in delirium as they may worsen symptoms and have been shown to be ineffective. Melatonin is a pineal hormone, used as an attempt to restore the circadian rhythm in ICU patients, and hence decrease the risk factors for delirium. Dexmedetomidine is a selective and highly potent α2 adrenergic receptor agonist. It is used in a similar fashion to clonidine. It has just gained licence for use in the UK.

King J, Gratrix A. Delirium in intensive care. *Contin Educ Anaesth Crit Care Pain* 2009; 9(5):144–147

D16

Answer: d.

This baby does not have a strong indication for performing the operation under a regional or local technique. Since he went home at 36 weeks gestational age, it is unlikely that he required significant invasive ventilatory support as a neonate. He has been well since he was discharged. In sick babies, the operation can be done under local or regional technique. It is preferable to avoid opioids in ex-premature infants due to the increased risk of apnoeic episodes.

The intravenous paracetamol dosage should be 7.5 mg/kg for babies that are less than 10 kg, maximum daily dose of less than 60 mg/kg per 24 hours.

It is important to ensure the total dosage required for bilateral field blocks does not exceed the safety limit. The duration of the spinal may not be sufficient for bilateral hernia repairs.

MHRA Drug Safety Update. Drug safety advice: Intravenous paracetamol (Perfalgan): risk of accidental overdose, especially in infants and neonates. 2010; **3**, (12, 2)

D17
Answer: b.

Pseudo-addiction describes pain behaviours when the pain problem is under-treated. In this case the patient is experiencing ongoing pain as she is not able to re-locate her hip, which would usually resolve the pain. Therefore, she sought to acquire higher doses of analgesia. This could be confused with addiction and/or tolerance. Addiction is a primary, chronic, neuro-biological disease, with genetic, psychosocial and environmental factors influencing its development and manifestations. It is characterized by behaviours that include one or more of the following: impaired control over drug use, compulsive drug use, continued use despite harm and craving. Tolerance is where exposure to a drug results in a diminution of the drug's effects over time. Physical dependence is a state whereby a withdrawal syndrome can be elicited by abrupt cessation, rapid dose reduction or administration of an antagonist.

Tordoff S, Ganty P. Chronic pain and prescription misuse. *Contin Educ Anaesth Crit Care Pain* 2010;**10**(5):158–161
Pain and Substance Abuse: Improving the Patient Experience. British Pain Society guidelines 2007. Sourced: http://www.britishpainsociety.org/pub_professional.htm

D18
Answer: e.

While b and c are true, they are not the main priorities. Getting hold of the transplant team may provide some useful information, it is not mandatory if assessment of graft function is deemed to be adequate. Assessment of graft function and detecting the complications of immunosuppressive therapy (which include steroid-related side effects, the development of opportunistic infections, nephrotoxicity with renal impairment and subsequent hypertension, hepatotoxicity and bone marrow suppression) are the most important aspects of preoperative assessment in these patients.

Steadman R. Anaesthesia for liver transplant surgery. *Anesthesiol Clin N Am* 2004; **22**: 687–711
Morgan GE, Mikhail MS. *Clinical Anesthesiology*, 4th edn. USA: McGraw-Hill, 2006, 797–801

D19
Answer: e.

The statements are all correct apart from e. The overall risk of an instrumental delivery in labour is about 1 in 14. This rises to about 1 in 7 following an epidural.

Obstetric Anaesthetists Association. *Pain Relief in Labour* 3rd edn, 2008

D20

Answer: d.

Assessing pain in children can be difficult. Self-reporting scales or behavioural scales may be used.

Self-reporting scales: The Wong Baker Faces scale shows six faces from happy to crying and the child is asked to choose which one best describes their pain. The Oucher scale involves the child pointing to a photograph of a child in pain. The Wong Baker scale is more reliable in children 8–12 years, the Oucher has been validated in children as young as three. The adolescent paediatric pain tool is used for children between 8 and 17 years. The linear (visual) analogue scale uses a 10-centimetre line, which shows a range from no pain to worst pain, and the patient marks their position on the line.

Behavioural pain scales rely on assessment of the child's (usually age 1–5 years) behaviour. Examples are the Toddler–Preschooler Postoperative Pain Scale (TPPPS), the Children's Hospital Eastern Ontario Pain Scale (CHEOPS) and the Face Legs Activity Cry Consolability (FLACC) Scale

In this case, the fracture should be immobilized with a plaster of Paris back slab as this is effective in reducing pain. At this stage, oral analgesia should be sufficient if the patient is not nauseous or vomiting. A 10-year-old boy is not likely to agree to have suppositories and these, along with intramuscular injections are not necessary. The administration of intravenous morphine by bolus or infusion may result in nausea, vomiting and respiratory depression. Entonox is a useful adjunct for short procedures such as for applying immobilization, but would not be suitable analgesia for the 2 hours (or more) that he needs to wait until surgery. Once he returns from surgery, we would expect the pain and analgesic requirements to be reduced. Any increase in pain should alert to possible compartment syndrome of the limb.

Royal College of Nursing. Clinical Practice Guideline. *The Recognition and Assessment of Acute Pain in Children.* September 2009.

Tasker R, McClure R, Acerini C. *Oxford Handbook of Paediatrics* 2008. Oxford: Oxford University Press, 992

D21

Answer: a.

Non-specific low back pain refers to back pain with symptoms such as stiffness and soreness for which it is not possible to find a cause of the pain. The National Institute for Health and Clinical Excellence (NICE) issued guidelines in 2009 relating to the management of non-specific lower back pain of between 6 weeks' and 12 months' duration. Their guidelines were as follows:

- Offer one of the following:
  - A structured exercise programme tailored to the person
  - A course of manual therapy, e.g. spinal manipulation
  - Acupuncture
- Offer a combined physical and psychological treatment programme for those who have received the above, or have a greater disability
- Refer for possible spinal fusion if pain still severe

The use of imaging in the absence of red flags is inappropriate as would be starting an anti-neuropathic pain medication.

National Institute for Health and Clinical Excellence. Low back pain. Early management of persistent non-specific low back pain. Clinical guideline 88. Issue date: May 2009

D22
Answer: d.

Sensitivity = True positives / (True positives + False negatives), the clinical test correctly identifies the sick patients with the disease

Specificity = True negatives / (True negatives + False positives), the test correctly identifies those patients who are not sick

Positive predictive value (PPV) = True positives / (True positives + False positives). It is also called the precision rate as it measures the proportion of patients who are correctly diagnosed when they test positive.

Negative predictive value (NPV) = True negatives / (True negatives + False negatives)

The likelihood ratio of a clinical test predicts the probability or the odds of having the disease when tested positive as compared with ones who test negative, i.e. = sensitivity / 1 − specificity.

Lalkhen AG, McCluskey A. Clinical tests: sensitivity and specificity. *Contin Educ Anaesth Crit Care Pain* 2008; 8(6): 221–223

D23
Answer: c.

In the management of a patient with aortic stenosis, the key concerns are to maintain a normal heart rate and rhythm, adequate systemic vascular resistance (SVR) and sufficient intravascular volume and venous return; in the face of a fixed stroke volume. Arterial blood pressure monitoring is indicated, and some anaesthetists advocate pulmonary artery catheterization as well to facilitate monitoring of fluid balance. Spinal anaesthesia is contra-indicated, due to the significant decrease in SVR that can occur. Epidural analgesia should be slowly titrated to allow appropriate compensatory fluid administration and vasoconstriction above the level of the block. The use of adrenaline should be avoided, as inadvertent intra-vascular injection can cause tachycardia. Hypovolaemia and decreased venous return (pre-load) are of much greater concern than pulmonary oedema, therefore the pulmonary artery wedge pressure should be maintained at high-normal levels in the range of 15–17 mmHg.

Chestnut, D, Polley LS, Tsen LC *et al. Chestnut's Obstetric Anesthesia: Principles and Practice*, 2009. Philadelphia: Elsevier Mosby

D24
Answer: a.

Acute poisoning is relatively common and is the cause of significant morbidity and mortality. Owing to the circumstances of where the poisoning occurred and the symptoms, it is most likely this presentation is due to ethylene glycol poisoning.

Ethylene glycol is a sweet-tasting liquid, which is why young children often consume it. The early presentation can look very similar to intoxication from alcohol. Patients present with a profound metabolic acidosis with a high anion gap. The metabolites of ethylene glycol can cause acute renal failure. Treatment includes ethanol, which competes for the enzyme (alcohol dehydrogenase) that metabolizes the ethylene glycol. Fomepizole blocks the metabolism of methanol and ethylene glycol and can be injected every 12 hours, but is expensive and not widely available. Haemodialysis is also helpful in ethylene glycol poisoning.

Ward C, Sair M. Oral poisoning: an update. *Contin Educ Anaesth Crit Care Pain* 2010; **10**(1): 6–11

D25

Answer: e.

CBF autoregulation is maintained with alpha-stat pH management. The other options are all consequences of DHCA. In adult aortic arch surgery the acid–base management of cardiopulmonary bypass is controversial. With a significant decrease in body core temperature, gases are more soluble in the blood and thus the pCO_2 decreases and pH increases. The addition of CO_2 to the circulation in the attempt to normalize blood pH (at the temperature of the patient) during DHCA deranges cerebral autoregulation, increases CBF and may increase embolic load. The alpha-stat approach aims to keep the pH neutral at blood corrected to 37 °C, and is tolerant of alkalosis at the patient's actual temperature. The 'alpha' in alpha-stat refers to the ionization state of imidazole groups of intracellular proteins; the rationale cited by the proponents of alpha-stat management is that the enzymatic processes and intra-cellular protein function are better maintained when this ionization state is kept physiological.

Conolly S. Deep hypothermic circulatory arrest. *Contin Educ Anaesth Crit Care Pain* 2010; **10**(5): 138–142

D26

Answer: d.

This is almost pulseless electrical activity, although continuing CO_2 suggests some circulation. Given the history, it is most likely that, following forceful insertion of the prosthesis into the shaft of femur, a fat embolism was created, which then lay in the femoral vein occluded by the leg position. When the leg was straightened and patency restored to the femoral vein, the embolus could then migrate. Bone cement reaction may exert a similar effect and is characterized by hypoxia, hypotension or both and/or unexpected loss of consciousness occurring around the time of cementation, prosthesis insertion, reduction of the joint or, occasionally, limb tourniquet deflation in a patient undergoing cemented bone surgery. This surgery was, however, uncemented.

Donaldson AJ. Bone cement implantation syndrome. *Br J Anaesth* 2009; **102**(1): 12–22

D27

Answer: e.

An absolute contra-indication to renal transplant would be active infection or malignancy. Patients are very often dehydrated, as they have frequently received recent dialysis. It is important therefore to assess fluid status and administer appropriate fluids to avoid hypotension, as it increases the chances of acute tubular necrosis in the graft. Delayed gastric emptying is common in patients with uraemia and H_2 antagonists should be given as a pre-med. A recent potassium result is essential prior to anaesthetic in patients with end-stage renal failure. This patient is anuric and the potassium can rise quickly, so a result within the preceding 6 hours is vital.

Rabey PG. Anaesthesia for renal transplantation. *Contin Educ Anaesth Crit Care Pain* 2001; 1: 24–27

D28
Answer: e.

In obese patients, the volume of the central compartment is unchanged, but the volume of distribution of the highly fat-soluble drugs like barbiturates increases greatly. For such drugs, the induction dose should be based on ideal body weight (IBW), as their peak plasma concentration is the same as when the dose is adjusted according to the patients cardiac output.

Propofol, despite being a highly fat-soluble drug is not dosed according to the IBW, but as per total body weight (TBW) as it has a very high clearance. At a steady state, its volume of distribution and clearance are relative to TBW. The same is true when using propofol infusions for TIVA.

Neuromuscular blocking drugs are water soluble and have a negligible change in the volume of distribution. Dosing by lean body weight (LBW) is more accurate (LBW = IBW + 20%). Suxamethonium doses, when used for rapid sequence, should be calculated according to the TBW as it ensures good conditions for intubation.

Local anaesthetics should be calculated as per the IBW due to the risk of toxicity at higher doses. When used neuraxially, the dose should be decreased by 25%. This is because the volume of the epidural space in the obese is reduced due to presence of excess fat and engorged veins. The appropriate dosing scale for most anaesthetic drugs including opioids in the obese is usually LBW.

Lotia S, Bellamy MC. Anaesthesia and morbid obesity. *Contin Educ Anaesth Crit Care Pain* 2008; **8**(5): 151–156
Ingrade J, Lemmens HJM. Dose adjustment of anaesthetics in the morbidly obese. *Br J Anaesth* 2010; **105**(Suppl 1): i16–i23

D29
Answer: d.

The current available guidelines concerned with the use of perioperative beta-blockers have been produced by the European Society of Cardiology (ESC) and the American College of Cardiology Foundation/American Heart Association (ACCF/AHA). These were updated following the results of the PeriOperative Ischemia Study Evaluation Trial (POISE), which showed that beta blockade reduced cardiac risk, but increased all-cause mortality and the risk of disabling stroke. The main points from these guidelines are:

- Chronic therapy with beta-blockers should be continued
- Beta-blockers should be titrated to heart rate 60–80 bpm with systolic pressure more than 100 mmHg (ESC) or *in the absence of hypotension* (ACCF/AHA).
- Should it be indicated, beta-blocker therapy should be started early, from days to weeks before surgery.
- High-cardiac-risk patients undergoing high-risk surgery, particularly vascular, are more likely to benefit than low-risk patients.

European Society of Cardiology. Guidelines for Pre-operative Cardiac Risk Assessment and Perioperative Cardiac Management in Non-cardiac Surgery. *Europ Heart J* 2009; **30**: 2769–2812

ACCF/AHA focused update on perioperative beta blockade. *J Am Coll Cardiol* 2009; 54:2102–2128

Sear JW, Foex P. Recommendations on perioperative β-blockers: differing guidelines: so what should the clinician do? *Br J Anaesth* 2010; **104**(3): 273–275

D30

Answer: c.

Although b and e are true, they should not be the *focus* of your preoperative assessment. Although the haematocrit is usually high or normal, it is not a *reliable* indicator of volume status. Premedication may be useful, but it is not essential. Ensuring an adequate post-operative bed is an essential part of their *whole* perioperative management, it is not the focus of your *preoperative* assessment. Evidence of end-organ damage (such as cerebral infarction, hypertensive encephalopathy, intracranial haemorrhage or subarachnoid haemorrhage, acute MI or unstable angina, acute pulmonary oedema and aortic dissection) should also be sought as part of your preoperative assessment.

Steadman R. Anaesthesia for liver transplant surgery. *Anesthesiology Clin N Am* 2004; **22**: 687–711

Morgan GE, Mikhail MS. Clinical Anesthesiology 4th edn, 2006. USA: McGraw-Hill, 797–801

Paper E – Questions

E1

A 55-year-old male with chronic obstructive pulmonary disease is undergoing LASER surgery. A flash of light is noticed, and the airway is thought to be on fire. The reading on the pulse oximeter is 90%.

Your first action is to:
a. Administer 100% oxygen and call for help
b. Administer steroids for airway oedema
c. Remove the endotracheal tube and assess the airway
d. Discontinue ventilation and disconnect oxygen
e. Flood the airway with sterile water

E2

A 49-year-old male is on coronary care. He has suffered an ST-elevation myocardial infarction. Primary percutaneous coronary intervention was unsuccessful for anatomical reasons, and he therefore underwent thrombolysis. He continues to have pain at rest, but without further ECG changes. On examination he is pale, clammy and peripherally cool. Blood pressure is 80/30 mmHg. The surgeons wish to have him transferred for stabilization and subsequent coronary artery bypass grafting.

He should now be considered for:
a. Repeat thrombolysis
b. Further angioplasty
c. Insertion of intra-aortic balloon pump
d. Adrenaline infusion
e. GTN infusion

E3

A 44-year-old lady is scheduled for pituitary tumour resection under general anaesthesia. Over the past few years she has noticed her hands have got larger and her hats no longer fit. She has been diagnosed with acromegaly.

Which of the following concurrent disorders is the patient most likely to exhibit?
a. Toxic thyroid goitre

Practice Single Best Answer Questions for the Final FRCA, ed. Hozefa Ebrahim, Khalid Hasan, Mark Tindall, Michael Clarke and Natish Bindal. Published by Cambridge University Press. © Cambridge University Press 2013.

b. Hypogonadism
c. Obstructive sleep apnoea
d. Impaired glucose tolerance
e. Hypertension

E4

Cardiopulmonary exercise testing is a reliable and objective test for assessing functional status prior to surgery. There are certain medical conditions, however, which are absolute contra-indications to undertaking the test.

Which of the following lists includes conditions which are all absolute contra-indications?
a. Resting saturations <85%, unstable angina, thyrotoxicosis, syncope
b. Hyperkalaemia, pregnancy, tachyarrythmias, cognitive impairment
c. Pulmonary oedema, hypertension, obesity, renal failure
d. Hypomagnesaemia, anaemia, schizophrenia, peripheral vascular disease
e. Pulmonary embolus, unstable angina, pregnancy, Turner's syndrome

E5

A 65-year-old male presents for emergency reduction of an incarcerated inguinal hernia. He has a history of resistant depression and is treated with phenelzine (a monoamine oxidase inhibitor). He receives 75 mg intravenous diclofenac and local anaesthetic infiltration to the wound intraoperatively. In recovery he complains of pain of moderate severity.

Which of the following would be the most appropriate analgesic option?
a. Tramadol 100 mg iv and paracetamol 1 g iv
b. Morphine 0.1 mg/kg iv
c. Pethidine 1 mg/kg iv and paracetamol 1 g iv
d. Tramadol 100 mg iv
e. Morphine 0.1 mg/kg iv and tramadol 100 mg iv

E6

You are anaesthetizing a patient for an appendiceal carcinoid tumour resection when the patient suddenly becomes profoundly flushed and hypotensive.

What would be the most appropriate therapy to stabilise the patient's physiology?
a. Adrenaline
b. Noradrenaline
c. Phenylephrine
d. Octreotide
e. Enoximone

E7

A 74-year-old male with long-standing Parkinson's disease requires a general anaesthetic for a laparoscopic-assisted hemicolectomy. He tells you that he has had a general anaesthetic two years ago and was 'unable to move' afterwards. He was unable to tell you what drugs he was given and you do not yet have access to his old notes.

Which of the following drugs may induce muscle rigidity in treated Parkinson's disease?
a. Metoclopramide

b. Pethidine
c. Amitriptyline
d. Cyclizine
e. Atropine

E8

Beta-blockers may be used in the management of high-risk patients in the perioperative period to reduce cardiac risk.

What is the main rationale behind this therapy?
a. To decrease myocardial oxygen consumption by reducing the heart rate
b. Redistribution of coronary flow to the subendocardium
c. Stabilisation of atheromatous plaques
d. An increase in the threshold for ventricular fibrillation
e. Better control of intraoperative blood pressure

E9

There are many ways to assess severity of aortic stenosis.

Which is the most accurate?
a. Peak-to-peak gradient by left heart catheter
b. Mean gradient by trans-thoracic echocardiography (TTE)
c. Aortic valve area calculated by continuity equation during TTE and indexed to body surface area
d. NYHA class
e. Loudness of heart murmur with the presence of a plateau pulse

E10

You are called to assist with a 17-year-old patient with Down syndrome having an appendicectomy. He is known to have a ventricular septal defect with Eisenmenger's syndrome and his saturations have dropped to 70% despite F_iO_2 of 100%.

The most appropriate intervention is to:
a. Give a fluid challenge
b. Add positive end-expiratory pressure
c. Increase ventilation
d. Give vasoconstrictors
e. Give prostacyclin

E11

You are asked to review a 55-year-old man in recovery following an uneventful, but prolonged, laparoscopic prostatectomy. He is acutely confused and has stridor. His past medical history includes hypertension, stable angina and a hiatus hernia. He had an uneventful general anaesthetic with transversus abdominis plane blocks and 10 mg of morphine intravenously.

What is the most likely cause for the confusion and stridor?
a. Local anaesthetic toxicity
b. Anaphylaxis

c. Urinary retention
d. CO_2 embolism
e. Cerebral and laryngeal oedema

E12

You are anaesthetizing a 4-year-old child for unilateral squint correction. Twenty minutes into the procedure, the child is breathing spontaneously on sevoflurane at a rate of 24 breaths per minute. Her heart rate drops to 40 bpm. You inform the surgeon, and ask her to stop operating.

The next appropriate action is:
a. Administer atropine 20 mcg/kg and ask the surgeons to reschedule the case for another day
b. Allow surgery to continue once her heart rate improves
c. Administer adrenaline 10 mcg/kg, then allow surgery to continue
d. Administer atropine 20 mcg/kg, then allow surgery to continue
e. Paralyse and ventilate the patient, then allow the surgeons to continue once the end-tidal carbon dioxide is within normal limits

E13

You are asked to anaesthetize a patient with known aortic stenosis for an orthopaedic procedure. Midway through the procedure the ECG changes from sinus rhythm to an irregular narrow complex tachycardia. The blood pressure drops.

The most important action would be to:
a. Administer vasopressors
b. Check electrolytes and correct any imbalances
c. Give a fluid bolus
d. Immediate cardioversion
e. Give 100% oxygen

E14

Pregnancy causes a hypercoagulable state.

Which of the following statements is most accurate?
a. Platelet count increases, with a maximal increase in the third trimester
b. Factors VII, VIII, X and XII increase during pregnancy, whilst von Willebrand factor decreases
c. Fibrinolysis is reduced in pregnancy due to an decrease in t-PA activity
d. Protein C and Protein S are decreased during pregnancy
e. D-Dimer levels decrease during pregnancy

E15

Regarding transdermal fentanyl preparations, which of the following statements is incorrect?
a. Fentanyl patches result in the formation of a fentanyl reservoir in the skin
b. Maximum plasma concentrations of fentanyl occur 12–24 h after patch application
c. Exposure to heat increases fentanyl delivery by up to one-third

d. Transdermal fentanyl can be used for acute pain control

e. Clarithromycin reduces the effectiveness of the fentanyl patch

E16

Gabapentin is an anticonvulsant commonly used as an agent to treat neuropathic pain.

Its mechanism of action is primarily due to effects at which of the following sites?

a. Calcium channels

b. $GABA_A$-receptors

c. $GABA_B$- receptors

d. NMDA-receptors

e. Sodium channels

E17

You are called to see a 5-year-old child in A&E who has respiratory distress. You note that she is stridulous, sitting in the upright position, drooling and using accessory muscles of respiration. She is febrile with a temperature of 39.5 °C.

Which of the following statements is correct?

a. The most likely diagnosis is moderately severe croup and she should be treated with oral dexamethasone and admitted overnight to a paediatric ward

b. The history fits with a diagnosis of epiglottitis and she should be immediately intubated in the resuscitation room with a rapid sequence induction

c. She should be transferred to PICU for monitoring, cannulation, bloods, fluids and antibiotics

d. She is likely to have inhaled a foreign body and should be sent for inspiratory and expiratory chest films, after which she should be transferred to theatre for removal of the foreign body

e. Her airway may be precarious and she should be transferred to theatre for intubation with an inhalational induction and avoidance of the use of muscle relaxants

E18

The obstetricians have admitted a woman with pre-eclampsia to the high dependency unit. You have been asked to review her.

Which of the following statements about pre-eclampsia is false?

a. A systolic blood pressure >170 mmHg on two occasions with proteinuria ≥+++ constitutes severe pre-eclampsia

b. Spinal anaesthesia is relatively contra-indicated

c. Magnesium may be given prior to intubation

d. Labetalol is the first-line treatment for management of hypertension

e. Eclampsia can present postnatally

E19

Which one of the following would be most appropriate for the treatment of portal hypertension?

a. Vasopressin

b. Octreotide

c. Bisoprolol
d. Propranolol
e. Sodium and water restriction

E20

A 54-year-old female presents to the pain clinic with a 2-month history of episodic, severe stabbing pains in the left cheek. It can be brought on by innocuous factors such as light touch. There are no autonomic features.

What is the most likely diagnosis?
a. Cluster headache
b. Trigeminal neuralgia
c. SUNCT (short-lasting, unilateral neuralgiform headaches with conjunctival tearing)
d. Paroxysmal hemicrania
e. Tempero-mandibular disorder

E21

A 9-month-old infant is brought into hospital by his parents with suspected meningitis. The paediatric registrar manages to site a cannula on the dorsum of his hand but is unable to obtain a blood sample. On examination, he is difficult to rouse, cool peripherally and has purpuric spots on his lower leg. His temperature has been measured at 39.5 °C

The next most appropriate action is:
a. Perform a lumbar puncture
b. Take blood cultures
c. Administer intravenous fluid bolus of 20 ml/kg
d. Administer iv paracetamol
e. Administer a dose of intravenous ceftriaxone

E22

You have just performed brainstem death tests on a patient with a poor grade subarachnoid haemorrhage. You have discussed organ donation with the family and the transplant co-ordinator is on their way. The nurse reports that she is having to increase the patient's nordrenaline infusion in order to maintain a MAP of 70 mmHg.

What is your next action?
a. Insert an oesophageal Doppler for cardiac output monitoring
b. Do not increase the current ICU support since it is not in the patient's best interests
c. Start vasopressin
d. Start tri-iodothyronine
e. Give methylpredisolone 15 mg/kg iv

E23

A 20-year-old cyclist is involved in a high-speed road traffic collision. On arrival to A&E, you note that he has some blood around his nose and mouth and you suspect a facial fracture. His respiratory rate is 12/min, but the pattern is irregular. The heart rate is 100/min and BP 100/40 mmHg. Glasgow Coma Score is 9/15 (E2 V2 M5), pupils equal and reactive to light. He had a brief, self-terminating generalized tonic–clonic seizure witnessed on his arrival to the department. An arterial blood gas analysis gives the following results: pO_2 12 kPa, pCO_2 6.0 kPa on 15l/min O_2 via face mask.

The next most important step in the management plan would be to:
a. Organize for transfer of the patient to a Level 1 Trauma centre with an anaesthetic escort
b. Load the patient with iv phenytoin
c. Transfer the patient immediately for a CT head
d. Intubate and ventilate immediately
e. Complete the secondary survey

E24

Acute lung injury (ALI) and acute respiratory distress syndrome (ARDS) are common in sick patients, particularly in those admitted to critical care units. Knowledge of the pathogenesis and treatment of these disorders is important in intensive care medicine.

Which of the following represents current knowledge of lung injury?
a. Cardiomegaly is generally not a feature of ARDS
b. The proliferative phase of ALI is accompanied by an increase in lung compliance
c. Pleural effusions are commonly seen in ALI
d. The acute phase of ALI includes eosinophilic alveolar infiltrates
e. Ventilation should be aimed at normalising blood gases

E25

A general surgeon asks your advice on the management of a patient with inoperable pancreatic carcinoma who is currently an outpatient. The patient has severe abdominal pain that has failed to respond to a combination of paracetamol, diclofenac and codeine.

Appropriate pain control interventions for this patient would *not* include?
a. Amitriptyline in escalating doses at night
b. Gabapentin in escalating doses three times daily
c. Oral morphine dosed according to pain
d. Training in the use of transcutaneous electrical nerve stimulation (TENS)
e. Admittance for a trial of thoracic epidural pain relief

E26

A 6-year-old child is booked for a tonsillectomy. The nurse informs you that they have been unable to weigh the child but have managed to perform some routine observations.

Which of the following is most consistent with a healthy 6-year-old at rest?
a. Weight 25 kg, Heart rate 100, Breaths per min 20
b. Weight 20 kg, Heart rate 100, Breaths per min 20
c. Weight 20 kg, Heart rate 70, Breaths per min 25
d. Weight 25 kg, Heart rate 70, Breaths per min 30
e. Weight 25 kg, Heart rate 110, Breaths per min 30

E27

A 46-year-old mechanic is referred to the chronic pain clinic. He has a 6-month history of altered sensation, pain and reduced function in his right hand. His general practitioner has diagnosed complex regional pain syndrome (CRPS). He has been prescribed amitriptyline, gabapentin and nifedipine, the pain has improved slightly and he is receiving no other treatment.

What treatment would you offer first at clinic today?
a. Prescribe 50% dimethyl sulfoxide cream
b. Offer a TENS machine and instruction in its use
c. Prescribe transdermal fentanyl
d. Offer intravenous guanethidine block
e. Request a course of physiotherapy

E28

A 56-year-old female is undergoing posterior fossa craniotomy in the sitting position for debulking of a clival tumour. Thirty minutes after commencement of surgery, there is an abrupt fall in end-tidal carbon dioxide concentration from 4.5 kPa to 2 kPa accompanied by an audible change in the precordial Doppler signal.

Which of the following interventions should be performed first?
a. Reposition the patient with the left side down
b. Administer an intravenous fluid bolus
c. Inform the surgeon and ensure the surgical field is covered with saline-soaked swabs
d. Aspirate immediately from the central venous catheter
e. Temporarily compress the patient's jugular veins

E29

Peripheral nerve blocks can often be used in place of neuraxial blocks, and may reduce the need for postoperative opiates and their accompanying side effects.

Which of the following is true?
a. Most operations on the foot can be performed under sciatic block
b. The saphenous nerve is a branch of the obturator nerve and supplies the medial area between the knee and the ankle
c. The sciatic nerve contains branches from L2–4 and S1–3
d. Clonidine is of no benefit in sciatic blocks
e. The Labat approach to the sciatic nerve requires the patient to be supine

E30

A 33-year-old previously healthy female with a history of moderate alcohol use presents to the Emergency Department with 2 weeks of abdominal pain, constipation, abdominal distension and jaundice. Blood results revealed abnormal liver function tests and deranged clotting. Paracentesis is performed; the neutrophil count is $330 \, mm^{-3}$.

The most likely diagnosis is:
a. Klinefelter syndrome
b. Perforated small bowel
c. Hepatitis C
d. Spontaneous bacterial peritonitis
e. Haemochromatosis

Paper E – Answers

E1

Answer: d.

Fire in the airway is a potential problem with LASER surgery. The management of such an occurrence would include the following:

- Disconnect oxygen and stop ventilation. This will only exacerbate the fire
- Irrigate the airway with sterile water if the fire persists
- Remove the burnt endotracheal tube
- Re-intubate and ventilate
- Assess the airway with a bronchoscope
- Assess the patient's need for additional therapies such as steroids and antibiotics depending on the clinical need.

Schramm VL Jr, Mattox DE, Stool SE. Acute management of laser-ignited intratracheal explosion. *Laryngoscope* 1981; **91**(9,1): 1417–1426

E2

Answer: c.

This patient has cardiogenic shock and ongoing coronary ischaemia without ECG changes. There is no indication for repeat thrombolysis on ECG criteria and the blood pressure is low. The treatment of choice is coronary artery bypass grafting. In order to stabilize the patient, placement of an intra-aortic balloon pump would increase coronary blood flow and reduce myocardial workload whilst augmenting the patient's blood pressure. This would hopefully result in resolution of the patient's symptoms and provide a period of stability.

An adrenaline infusion may improve blood pressure but would have the effect of increasing myocardial workload and the resultant tachycardia would compromise coronary blood flow, so would not be the treatment of choice in this setting.

The patient is too hypotensive to receive a GTN infusion.

Krishna M, Zacharowski K. Principles of intra-aortic balloon pump counterpulsation. *Contin Educ Anaesth Crit Care Pain* 2009; **9**(1): 24–28

Practice Single Best Answer Questions for the Final FRCA, ed. Hozefa Ebrahim, Khalid Hasan, Mark Tindall, Michael Clarke and Natish Bindal. Published by Cambridge University Press. © Cambridge University Press 2013.

E3

Answer: b.

This lady has a growth hormone-secreting pituitary tumour that is causing acromegaly.

In acromegaly benign thyroid goitre may be present in 30%–90% of patients; however, the incidence of toxic goitre is much less. Patients may report symptoms of obstructive sleep apnoea. While this is common in acromegalic patients as a group, it is much less common in women than in men. Impaired glucose tolerance may be present in up to 45% of cases with frank diabetes being slightly less.

Hypogonadism may be present in greater than 50% of patients; a result of concomitant hyperprolactinaemia or gonadotrophin insufficiency.

Memergut EC, Dumont AS, Barry UT, *et al*. Perioperative management of patients undergoing transsphenoidal pituitary surgery. *Anesth Analg* 2005; **101**: 1170–1181

Scacchi M, Cavagnini F. Acromegaly. *Pituitary* 2006; **9**: 297–303

E4

Answer: a.

Resting saturations <85%, unstable angina, thyrotoxicosis and syncope are all **absolute** contra-indications to cardiopulmonary exercise testing. Pulmonary oedema and cognitive disorders, if they impact on understanding, are also absolute contra-indications. Relative contra-indications include electrolyte abnormalities, advanced or complex pregnancy, tachyarrythmias and pulmonary hypertension. Cardiopulmonary exercise testing is likely to be of benefit in assessing those patients with hypertension, obesity, renal failure and peripheral vascular disease.

Agnew N. Preoperative cardiopulmonary exercise testing. *Contin Educ Anaesth Crit Care Pain* 2010; **10**(2): 33–37

E5

Answer: b.

Monoamine oxidase inhibitors (MAOI) such as phenelzine, tranylcypromine and isocarbox-azid are antidepressants used, rarely, in the treatment of refractory depression. Their continuation in the perioperative period is of concern to the anaesthetist because of their propensity for drug interactions. There are two main types of drug reaction: hypertensive crises and the serotonin syndrome, both of which can be fatal.

Hypertensive crises may be precipitated by the co-administration of MAOIs and indirectly acting sympathomimetics such as ephedrine. Since ephedrine is metabolized by monoamine oxidases, it may cause an exaggerated response in such patients.

The serotonin syndrome is characterized by three groups of excitatory phenomena:

- *muscular hyperactivity* including clonus, tremor and hyperreflexia
- *autonomic hyperactivity* including tachycardia, pyrexia and diaphoresis
- *agitation and confusion.*

It is caused by the co-administration of MAOIs and serotonin reuptake inhibitors, for example, tricyclic antidepressants, SSRIs, and serotonin and noradrenaline reuptake inhibitors (SNRIs).

Some opioid analgesics have weak serotonin reuptake inhibitor actions. Case reports of serotonin toxicity exist for co-administration with MAOIs of pethidine, tramadol and dextromethorphan. These should be avoided in such patients. Morphine, fentanyl, codeine and remifentanil all appear to be safe.

Paracetamol is safe in this case.

Gillman PK. Monoamine oxidase inhibitors, opioid analgesics and serotonin toxicity. *Br J Anaesth* 2005; **95**: 434–441

E6

Answer: d.

Carcinoid tumours are derived from enterochromaffin cells and secrete peptides and amines, many of which are vasoactive. Most tumours are located within the GI tract (75%), but may also develop in the bronchi, pancreas or gonads. Vasoactive mediators include serotonin, histamine, substance P, vasoactive intestinal peptide and prostaglandins. When released into the systemic circulation, these can produce the 'carcinoid syndrome' with flushing, labile blood pressure, diarrhoea and bronchospasm. Most carcinoid tumours drain into the portal venous system and so the liver metabolizes the hormones before systemic effects can result. Only tumours which have metastasized or are located outside this system produce the effects listed above. The syndrome can be triggered by particular foods (tyramine in cheese), the handling of tumours, stress and catecholamine/histamine release. Octreotide produces pharmacological actions similar to the endogenous hormone somatostatin. It reduces the secretion of serotonin, as well as other hormones, from carcinoid tumours and is useful in reversing the effects of the carcinoid syndrome. It is used to stabilize patients' physiology prior to operating and it can be used in 20–100 mcg boluses iv intraoperatively. Noradrenaline and adrenaline, being catecholamines, have classically been avoided during carcinoid crises as they may activate kallikrein within the tumour. This results in release of bradykinin, which may paradoxically worsen hypotension. Phenylephrine is more often used for control of hypotension (resistant to octreotide) in these patients, once other causes for hypotension have been excluded. Enoximone may be useful in those patients who have cardiac disease associated with carcinoid (right-sided valve disease and fibrosis) to increase cardiac output, but it must be borne in mind that it will worsen peripheral dilatation and so should not be the first-line therapy in the example above.

Powell BA, Mukhtar A, Mills GH. Carcinoid: the disease and its implications for anaesthesia. *Contin Educ Anaesth Crit Care Pain* 2011; **11**(1): 9–13

E7

Answer: b.

There are many drug interactions involving those used for treating Parkinson's disease. Those of particular relevance are discussed below.

- Opiates are often necessary after major surgery, but may worsen muscle rigidity (it is likely that the amount of morphine used for analgesia is far less than this). Pethidine should be avoided as it can cause hypertension and muscle rigidity in patients on selegiline, but will not cause extra-pyramidal side effects.

- Antidepressants – the use of TCAs may potentiate levodopa-induced arrhythmias.
- Antipsychotics (e.g. phenothiazines, butyrophenones, piperazine derivatives) may worsen PD symptoms; it is best to use atypical antipsychotics (e.g.sulpiride, clozapine).
- Anti-hypertensive agents may cause severe hypotension in those with PD (due to postural hypotension, hypovolaemia).
- Volatile agents: the use of halothane can potentiate levodopa-induced arrhythmias.
- iv induction agents – propofol may have dopamine-like effects, and thus help reduce tremor and muscle rigidity.
- Anticholinergic drugs – centrally acting ones (e.g. atropine) can precipitate central anticholinergic syndrome. Glycopyrrolate is the anticholinergic of choice.
- Antiemetics are of importance, as nausea/vomiting can hinder restarting enteral PD drugs. Antiemetics deemed unsafe to use in PD are metoclopramide, droperidol and prochlorperazine, as these drugs will worsen PD symptoms and cause extrapyramidal effects. The antiemetic of choice is domperidone. 5-HT3 anatagonists (e.g. ondansetron, granisetron) can be used in patients with PD. The use of antihistamine anti-emetics (e.g. cyclizine) is also safe.

Errington DR, Severn AM, Meara J. Parkinsons disease. *Contin Educ Anaesth Crit Care Pain* 2002; 2: 69–73

E8

Answer: a

The use of beta-blockers in the perioperative period provides a number of cardio-protective effects including redistribution of coronary blood flow to the subendocardium, plaque stabilization and an increase in the threshold for VF. However, the main rationale is to decrease myocardial oxygen consumption by controlling heart rate and decreasing myocardial contractility.

European Society of Cardiology. Guidelines for preoperative cardiac risk assessment and perioperative cardiac management in non-cardiac surgery. *Europ Heart J* 2009; 30: 2769–2812

E9

Answer c.

Aortic valve area is the best method. Gradients may be affected by LV systolic function such that the gradients across a stenotic valve will reduce as the ventricle begins to fail. A high gradient is suggestive of a tight valve (and the ability of the LV to generate sufficient pressure), but a low gradient may indicate impending LV failure. Symptoms and signs may be misleading as the patient adjusts to a more limited exercise capacity, avoiding activities that precipitate symptoms such as pre-syncope, chest tightness and shortness of breath. The valve area – the orifice area – is what matters and constitutes the afterload against which the LV must generate work.

Brown J. Aortic stenosis and non-cardiac surgery. *Contin Educ Anaesth Crit Care Pain* 2005; 5(1): 1–4

E10

Answer: d.

Eisenmenger's syndrome exists when there is a persistent communication between the systemic and pulmonary circulations. This initially increases the pulmonary blood flow, but gives rise to pulmonary hypertension. Once the pulmonary pressures exceed systemic pressures, a right-to-left shunt results. This causes mixing of deoxygenated and oxygenated blood and results in cyanosis.

Any increases in pulmonary vascular resistance (PVR) or decreases in systemic vascular resistance (SVR) will worsen the right-to-left shunt. General anaesthesia will result in a drop in SVR, so this should anticipated and prevented. Metaraminol or noradrenaline can be used to maintain SVR, although they may also increase PVR to some extent.

Other factors that may increase PVR should also be controlled. These include:

- Hypoxia
- Hypercarbia
- Histamine
- Low lung volumes
- Nitrous oxide

Other treatments for chronic pulmonary hypertension include pulmonary vasodilator therapies such as:

- Prostacyclin
- Bosentan (an endothelin receptor antagonist)
- Sildenafil

El-Chami MF, Searles CD. Eisenmenger syndrome: treatment and medication (online) Available at: http://emedicine.medscape.com/article/154555-treatment

E11

Answer: e.

Laparoscopic surgery has become increasingly popular due to its many benefits such as less postoperative pain, quicker recovery times and lower infection rates. Despite this, it should be remembered that laparoscopic surgery is not without its risks. The risks of laparoscopic surgery are either related to individual techniques and positioning or due to the physiological changes associated with the generation of a pneumoperitoneum.

Patient positioning is determined by the view that the surgeon is trying to optimize and often requires the extremes of the Trendelenburg or reverse Trendelenburg position with significant physiological effects. This particular problem is also compounded by the fact that many laparoscopic procedures can take significantly longer than their open equivalent.

Prolonged steep Trendelenburg position increases the risk of cerebral oedema, in addition to the risk associated with pneumoperitoneum, and upper airway oedema, which can present with transient stridor and confusion postoperatively. Compartment syndrome is also a rare but devastating complication caused by impaired arterial perfusion to raised lower limbs, compression of venous vessels by leg supports and reduced femoral venous drainage due to pneumoperitoneum.

The reverse Trendelenburg position results in reduced venous return, leading to hypotension and, potentially, myocardial and cerebral ischaemia.

Hayden P, Cowman S. Anaesthesia for laparoscopic surgery. *Contin Educ Anaesth Crit Care Pain* 2011; **11** (5): 177–180

E12

Answer: d.

The child presenting for squint surgery may be otherwise fit and well or may have associated diseases such as cerebral palsy, hydrocephalus, myopathies or other chromosomal abnormalities. Attention should be paid to these at the preoperative visit.

It is well known that strabismus surgery is associated with oculocardiac reflex. This is a bradycardic response to traction on any of the extraocular eye muscles (more commonly the medial rectus), which may also result in sinus arrest or major dysrhythmias. Afferent pathways are via the occipital branch of the trigeminal nerve and the efferent is via the vagus. Oculocardiac reflex occurs in approximately 60% of children undergoing squint surgery. On removal of traction the bradycardia resolves almost instantaneously. Prevention will involve administering atropine 20 mcg/kg, which may be given at induction as a routine or following a reflex event in theatre.

Most cases are anaesthetized with the child spontaneously breathing, but it should be noted that light anaesthesia or hypercarbia increases the risk of oculocardiac reflex.

Strabismus surgery is associated with significant postoperative nausea and vomiting (PONV), which may be linked to oculocardiac reflex since children who have bradycardias intraoperatively are at increased risk of PONV. Multimodal antiemetic prophylaxis should be administered.

The incidence of malignant hyperthermia is increased in patients with squint (still rare) but vigilance should be high.

James, I. Anaesthesia for paediatric eye surgery. *Contin Educ Anaesth Crit Care Pain* 2008; 8(1): 5–10

E13

Answer: d.

The principles of anaesthetizing a patient with aortic stenosis are:

- Maintain SVR with α-agonists in order to maintain coronary perfusion pressure and therefore myocardial oxygen supply. Not β-agonists as tachycardia should be avoided.
- Maintain normal sinus rhythm and promptly treat any arrhythmias.
- Avoid tachycardias which would reduce coronary artery filling time and reduce myocardial oxygenation.
- Maintain cardiac output to optimize intravascular volume and avoid extreme bradycardias.

In this question it is essential to restore sinus rhythm, and as the patient is already anaesthetized, cardioversion is the best option. The other measures would be beneficial but definitive treatment is necessary.

Brown J. Morgan-Hughes NJ. Aortic stenosis and non-cardiac surgery. *Contin Educ Anaesth Crit Care Pain* 2005; 5: 1–4

E14

Answer: c.

Platelet count decreases in normal pregnancy, due to increased destruction and haemodilution. von Willebrand factor increases in pregnancy, as well as factors VII, VIII, X, XII and ristocetin co-factor. Protein C levels remain the same or slightly increase. Protein S decreases. D-dimer levels increase, probably originating from the uterus.

Thornton P, Douglas J. Coagulation in pregnancy. *Best Pract Res Clin Obst Gynaecol* 2010; 24:339–352

E15

Answer: e.

Fentanyl is ideally suited for transdermal delivery. It is a lipophilic, small, and uncharged molecule, and so diffuses across the barrier of the skin well. It is also potent, so it is only required in low doses for good effect. It is being used increasingly in the chronic pain setting with 12/25/50/75/100 mcg/h release preparations available. The 12 mcg/h patch is roughly equivalent to 30–60 mg of oramorph over 24 h, and the 100 mcg/h preparation matches as much as 300–400 mg of oramorph over that time period. A standard fentanyl patch is applied to the skin for 72 hours. Each new patch requires around 12–24 h for peak drug concentrations to develop, but previous patches generate a reservoir of drug within the skin providing prolonged effect after patch removal. New devices that use iontophoresis (an electrical charge is used to increase drug movement transdermally) have incorporated fentanyl. Fentanyl patch PCAs have shown promise for acute pain control. Pharmacological interactions can affect the drug levels of fentanyl. Inhibitors of the enzyme CYP3A4, responsible for the metabolism of fentanyl, will prolong the action of fentanyl, possibly causing respiratory depression. These include clarithromycin, ketoconazole, amiodarone and the rate-limiting calcium channel blockers diltiazem and verapamil.

Bajaj S, Whiteman A, Brandner B *et al*. Transdermal drug delivery in pain management. *Contin Educ Anaesth Crit Care Pain* 2011; 11(2): 39–43

E16

Answer: a.

Gabapentin was designed as an antiepileptic medication and is used to control seizures, in particular partial seizures. Although structurally related to gamma amino-butyric acid (GABA), gabapentin does not bind to either of its receptors. Gabapentin (and pregabalin) binds to voltage-gated calcium channels at a particular subunit, the α_2-δ subunit. This interaction inhibits neurotransmitter release and this is where its use as an agent for neuropathic pain management originates. It has few interactions and is generally well tolerated, but side-effects, particularly when first started, are not uncommon. These include sedation and dizziness and the drug is sometimes started as a single night-time dose because of this. Gabapentin follows non-linear pharmacokinetics and dosing is usually divided into three;

starting at a low dose and increasing over a number of weeks to a maximum or until side effects become a problem.

Ballie JK, Power I. The mechanism of action of gabapentin in neuropathic pain. *Curr Opin Investig Drugs* 2006; 7(1): 33–39

E17

Answer: e.

Stridor is a high-pitched sound occurring as a result of turbulent airflow in the upper airways. It may be inspiratory, expiratory or biphasic. The most common causes of acute stridor are croup, foreign body and epiglottitis.

Croup is a general term referring to viral *laryngotracheitis* (parainfluenza virus), the non-infective *spasmodic croup* and *bacterial tracheitis* (*Staphylococcus aureus, Haemophilus influenzae*, streptococci, and Neisseria species). Croup usually affects children between the ages of 1 and 4 years and in most cases (with the exception of bacterial tracheitis) is self-limiting. Bacterial tracheitis usually necessitates intubation and ventilation and there are significant amounts of purulent debris and inflammatory pseudomembranes, which may obstruct the airways.

Inhalation of foreign body often has a clear history of choking or gagging. The severity of symptoms and the degree of airway obstruction will dictate the urgency with which surgery must be performed.

Epiglottitis is a medical emergency, and may be caused by *Haemophilus influenzae* type B, *Streptococcus pneumonia* and type A β-haemolytic streptococci. Epiglottitis presents with rapid onset of symptoms of high fever, dyspnoea, painful throat and a sensation of fullness in the throat. Speech and swallowing become difficult and the child appears quiet, anxious, drooling and toxic. As it progresses, the child will attempt to maximize air entry by sitting forward in the 'tripod' position and by extending the neck.

Management involves keeping the child calm and using an inhalational induction to gain control of the airway. This should be performed in theatre if possible. It is imperative to have access to a range of smaller endotracheal tubes, difficult airway equipment and an experienced ENT surgeon ready to perform an urgent tracheostomy if required. Usual choice of tube will be 0.5–1.0 mm (ID) smaller than expected for that aged child. Following intubation, laryngeal and blood cultures should be taken and extended spectrum cephalosporins commenced.

Maloney E, Meakin G. Acute stridor in children. *Contin Educ Anaesth Crit Care Pain* 2007; 7(6): 183–186

E18

Answer: b.

There are numerous definitions of severe pre-eclampsia. The MAGPIE trial described it as 'a DBP >110 mmHg on two occasions; or a SBP >170 mmHg on two occasions with proteinuria >3+; or a BP>150/100 mmHg on two occasions with proteinuria >2+ and at least two signs or symptoms of imminent eclampsia'.

There has been controversy about the use of spinal anaesthesia in preference to epidural anaesthesia. However, recent studies have shown that blood pressure changes in pre-eclamptic patients following spinal anaesthesia are less than in normotensive patients and no differences in neonatal Apgar scores or umbilical artery pH between the two techniques.

There may be an exaggerated pressor response to intubation, which may lead to stroke, cardiac dysrhythmias and pulmonary oedema. This may be minimized by alfentanil 10 mcg/kg 2 minutes prior to induction. (The paediatrician should always be informed if alfentanil is used.) Alternatives are magnesium sulphate 30–40 mg/kg, lignocaine 1.5 mg/kg or labetalol increments of 5 mg up to 15 mg.

Hydralazine has recently been displaced as drug of choice for management of hypertension. Up to 44% of eclampsia has been reported to occur postnatally.

The Magpie Trial Collaborative Group. Do women with pre-eclampsia, and their babies, benefit from magnesium sulphate? The Magpie Trial: a randomised placebo-controlled trial. *Lancet* 2002; **359**: 1877–1890

Visalyaputra S, Rodanant O, Somboonviboon W, Tantivitayatan K, Thienthong S, Saengchote W. Spinal versus epidural anesthesia for cesarean delivery in severe pre-eclampsia: a prospective randomized, multicenter study. *Anesth Analg* 2005; **101**(3): 862–868

E19

Answer: d.

Portal hypertension is defined as a portal pressure >10 mmHg. It is associated with the development of a collateral venous circulation, ascites and splenomegaly. The presence of gastric and oesophageal varices risks massive GI bleeding. A large amount of ascites leads to increased intra-abdominal pressure with a negative effect on respiratory and renal function. Splenomegaly leads to sequestration of platelets and thrombocytopenia.

Reduction of portal pressure is believed to reduce the formation of new blood vessels and development of the above complications. The drug of choice for treatment of portal hypertension is a non-cardioselective β-blocker such as propranolol or carvedilol.

Vasopressin and octreotide are used in the treatment of GI bleeding and ascites is treated with sodium and water restriction.

Vaja R, McNicol L, Sisley I. Anaesthesia for patients with liver disease. *Contin Educ Anaesth Crit Care Pain* 2010; **10**(1): 15–19

E20

Answer: b.

This may appear an easy question, but distinguishing trigeminal neuralgia from other similar differential diagnoses is a fundamental clinical skill.

This patient's symptoms and signs are typical of classic trigeminal neuralgia. The causes of headache and facial pain are numerous, but it is the specific features of trigeminal neuralgia as described above that make it easily diagnosed with a careful pain history. Cluster headache usually affects males with attacks lasting for weeks or months between pain-free periods. SUNCT (short-lasting, unilateral neuralgiform headaches with conjunctival tearing) is commonly mistaken for trigeminal neuralgia but is differentiated by its autonomic features, usually conjunctival tearing and injection. Paroxysmal hemicranias resemble cluster headaches though attacks are of shorter duration and more frequent (lasting 8–25 minutes and occurring 5–24 times a day). Temporomandibular disorder is a generic term used to describe a heterogenous range of disorders that involve continuous pain related to the masticatory muscles and/or the temporomandibular joint (TMJ). Limited mouth opening, bruxism and locking of the TMJ may also occur.

Zakrzewska JM. *Orofacial Pain*, 1st edn. Oxford: Oxford University Press, 2009

International Headache Society. The International Classification of Headache Disorders. *Cephalalgia* 2005; **24**(S1): 9–160

E21

Answer: e.

The most important thing is to give antibiotics and this should not be delayed by obtaining blood cultures or other investigations. It is also necessary to exclude raised intracranial pressure or coagulopathy before doing a lumbar puncture. In this case, he has an altered conscious level and a purpuric rash. Whole blood PCR testing for *Neisseria meningitidis* should be performed as soon as possible.

NICE guideline CG102 *Bacterial Meningitis and Meningococcal Septicaemia: Management of Bacterial Meningitis and Meningococcal Septicaemia in Children and Young People Younger than 16 Years in Primary and Secondary Care*. June 2010

E22

Answer: a.

Physiological changes occurring during the development of brainstem death may lead, if untreated, to rapid deterioration and cardiac arrest. The management of the brainstem dead donor is directed at restoring stability and to maintain or improve organ function in order to enhance the likelihood of successful transplantation.

Around the time of brainstem death, there can be a 'Cushing response' with dramatic cardiovascular changes. Following this, there can be a variable intensity and duration of 'sympathetic storm' with tachycardia, vasoconstriction and blood pressure instability. A later consequence is marked vasodilation and relative hypovolaemia; this is often due to fluid losses caused by the development of diabetes insipidus. Appropriate cardiovascular goals such as HR 60–100 bpm, CVP <12 mmHg, MAP 60–80 mmHg, cardiac index >2.4l/min per m², mixed venous oxygen saturation >60% should be aimed for.

In terms of management, the first priority is to restore an effective circulating volume with either colloid or crystalloid. Failure to promptly respond to appropriate fluid administration should mandate the use of more advanced cardiac output monitoring. The most effective vasopressor in this case is vasopressin and this may also treat diabetes insipidus if it has developed. If inotropic support is also required, then tri-iodothyronine (T3) or a catecholamine infusion should be considered.

A dose of 15 mg/kg of intravenous methyprednisolone is recommended once brainstem death is confirmed. Methylprednisolone use is associated with reduced lung water and therefore renders the lungs more suitable for transplant. Steroids may also ameliorate the process by which brainstem death itself increases the immunogenicity of solid organs increasing the risk of acute rejection in the recipient.

Edgar P, Bullock R, Bonner S. Management of the potential heart-beating donor. *Contin Educ Anaesth Crit Care Pain* 2004; **4**(3): 86–90

www.uktransplant.org.uk

E23

Answer: d.

In this situation, the mechanism of injury and the presentation all point towards a significant head injury. Worrying features include: likely soiled airway, possible complex unstable facial fracture, recurrent seizure activity and reduced Glasgow Coma Score (GCS). However, the clinical feature that determines his immediate management is the inadequate ventilation. He has an abnormal pattern of respiration and the ABG shows relative hypoxaemia and hypercarbia on high-flow oxygen therapy. The priority is to secure the airway in order to adequately ventilate the patient in the presence of a serious head injury. An increasing, uncontrolled, unmonitored $p\mathrm{CO_2}$ will lead to a potentially increased ICP and reduced cerebral perfusion pressure.

The other options are required, but will come once the most immediate threat to life has been managed. NICE Guidelines published for the management of head injury state that patients presenting with: coma (GCS $\leq$ 8), loss of protective laryngeal reflexes, ventilatory insufficiency (hypoxaemia ($P_a\mathrm{O_2}$ < 13 kPa on oxygen) or hypercarbia ($P_a\mathrm{CO_2}$ > 6 kPa); spontaneous hyperventilation causing $P_a\mathrm{CO_2}$ < 4 kPa or irregular respirations should be intubated and ventilated immediately.

Those presenting with a significantly deteriorating conscious level (1 or more points on motor score), unstable fractures of the facial skeleton, copious bleeding into mouth or seizures should be intubated and ventilated prior to transfer to a neurosurgical centre. Hypotension *per se* is not an indication for immediate intubation. Phenytoin should be given (after confirming with the neurosurgical team) to prevent further seizure activity. Finally, the secondary survey should only be completed once the primary survey has been satisfactorily completed and the most life-threatening problems addressed.

NICE Guidelines 2007. *Head Injury: Triage, Assessment, Investigation and Early Management of Head Injury in Infants, Children and Adults.* (http://www.nice.org.uk/nicemedia/live/11836/36257/36257.pdf)

E24

Answer: a.

Acute lung injury (ALI) is a poorly understood syndrome characterized by non-cardiogenic pulmonary oedema and respiratory failure in the presence of critical illness. Cardiomegaly does not necessarily preclude the diagnosis, but cardiac causes are more likely in the presence of LV dysfunction. ALI is divided into three phases.

- The *acute*, or exudative phase is characterized by hypoxaemia, and reduced lung compliance together with a lymphocytic alveolar infiltrate.

- The *subacute* or proliferative phase is characterized by continuing hypoxaemia and reduced lung compliance accompanied by proliferation of type-2 pneumocytes and formation of microvascular thrombus.
- The *proliferative* phase can either resolve with accompanying clinical improvement or can progress into the fibrotic stage, characterized by fibrotic changes and a loss of normal lung architecture. This may be accompanied by an improvement in oxygenation but is often associated with a reduction in CO_2 removal.

Several trials have assessed different ventilation strategies. The optimal strategy is a source of dispute, but results have been improved by using lower tidal volumes accompanied by higher PEEP and by accepting higher pCO_2 as long as acid–base balance is not grossly deranged.

Mahajan RP. Acute lung injury: options to improve oxygenation. *Contin Educ Anaesth Crit Care Pain* 2005; **5**(2): 52–55

Moloney ED, Griffiths MJD. Protective ventilation of patients with acute respiratory distress syndrome. *Br J Anaesth* 2004; **92**(2): 261–270

E25

Answer: a.

Cancer pain, especially in the retroperitoneum, will have a significant neuropathic component that may be addressed by amitriptyline and gabapentin. Amitriptyline should be started first due to the low cost of the drug and prominent secondary analgesic activity. Morphine will be required for acute pain control and later for breakthrough pain when slow release morphine is added. TENS may be effective and should be tried. The thoracic epidural should be reserved as an option if subcutaneous PCA should prove ineffective.

Vargas-Schaffer G. Is the WHO analgesic ladder still valid? Twenty-four years of experience. *Can Fam Physician* 2010; **56**: 514–517

E26

Answer: a.

The recommended methods of estimation of a child's weight include the use of population growth charts, Sandell or Broselow tapes and formulae. Which formulae to use has been subject of much debate. Over the last 20 years the formula for the calculation of weights of children aged 1–10 has traditionally been ([age + 4] x 2). However, over the same period of time, the weights of children in richer countries has generally increased and so this traditional formulae of ([age + 4] x 2) is thought to under-estimate weights, especially for older children. The formula ([age x 3] + 7) is now considered better for older children, although this can over-estimate weights for smaller children. The advanced life support group (ALGS) have recommended the following formulae:

Children aged 1–5: ([age $\times$ 2] + 8)
Children 6–10: ([age $\times$ 3] + 7)

Below is a table for expected heart and respiratory rates for varying ages.

Age (years)	Respiratory rate (breaths/min)	Heart rate (bpm)
<1	30–40	110–160
1–2	25–35	100–150
2–5	25–30	95–140
5–12	20–25	80–120
>12	15–20	60–100

Samuels M, Wieteska S eds. *Advanced Paediatric Life Support, The Practical Approach*, 5th edn. 2011. Advanced Life Support Group. London: Wiley-Blackwell

E27

Answer: e.

Dimethyl sulphoxide (DMSO) can be used for patients in an acute stage of the disease process where there is evidence of tissue oedema. DMSO acts to reduce the production of hypoxia-related oxygen free radicals. The prescription of opiates in CRPS is controversial and should not be undertaken without discussion with his GP.

TENS may be of benefit in neuropathic pain, but evidence for its use in CRPS is not strong.

Intravenous regional analgesia (IVRA) using agents such as lidocaine, clonidine, guanethidine, reserpine, and bretylium has been described. Randomized controlled trials have shown that IVRA is no better than placebo.

Physiotherapy is of benefit in maintaining and improving limb function and preventing secondary atrophy. The earlier it is commenced the better. It should be goal-directed and implemented such as to not aggravate the pain. This should be one of the first interventions offered.

Wilson JG, Serpell MG. Complex regional pain syndrome. *Contin Educ Anaesth Crit Care Pain* 2007; 7(2): 51–54

E28

Answer: c.

Posterior fossa surgery in the sitting position is associated with the risk of venous air embolism (VAE). It is caused by the ingress of air into open posterior fossa veins or venous sinuses situated above the level of the heart. The incidence of VAE in posterior fossa surgery has been estimated at 25%–50% when precordial Doppler is used.

The initial treatment priority in VAE is preventing the further entrainment of air, therefore communication with the operating surgeon and ensuring flooding of the operative site is essential. Other initial steps should proceed as follows:

- Increase F_iO_2 to 1.0
- Lower patient's head to raise venous pressure
- Attempt aspiration of air from a right atrial catheter where present
- Consider jugular venous compression
- Intravenous fluids or inotropes where required
- Cardiopulmonary resuscitation where appropriate

- Consider positioning left side down to ensure air remains in the right atrium

Matta BF, Menon DK, Turner JM (eds). *Textbook of Neuroanaesthesia and Critical Care.* London: Greenwich Medical Media, 2000
Porter J, Pidgeon C, Cunningham A. The sitting position in neurosurgery: a critical appraisal. *Br J Anaesth* 1999; **82**: 117–128

E29
Answer: a.

In the majority of patients the sciatic nerve supplies the lateral aspect of the leg below the knee and most of the foot. In about 10% of individuals the saphenous nerve supplies a portion of the foot below the medial malleolus and must therefore be blocked if operating on this area. The saphenous nerve is a branch of the femoral nerve. It supplies the medial cutaneous area below the knee. The sciatic nerve is composed of branches from L4–5 and S1–3 and provides the majority of innervation below the knee. Clonidine increases the duration of peripheral nerve blocks by 3 to 4 hours with minimal sedative effects.

In order to block the sciatic nerve using Labat's approach, the patient must be semi-prone with both hip and knee flexed.

Al-Haddad MF, Coventry DM. Major nerve blocks of the lower limb. *Contin Educ Anaesth Crit Care Pain* 2003; **3**(4): 102–105

E30
Answer: d.

The most likely diagnosis, given the history of alcohol excess, is alcoholic liver disease resulting in portal hypertension, ascites and a spontaneous bacterial peritonitis. This is confirmed by the elevated ascitic neutrophil count. Klinefelter syndrome can be associated with abdominal pain, but the syndrome is only seen in men. The history and the other signs and symptoms do not exclude small bowel perforation or hepatitis C, but they are less likely. Haemochromatosis whilst a definite cause of cirrhosis and ascites is unusual in females before the age of 50. The median age of onset in females is 66 and in males 51.

Jackson P, Gleeson D. Alcoholic liver disease. *Contin Educ Anaesth Crit Care Pain* 2010; **10**(3): 66–71

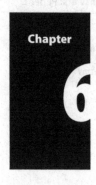

Chapter 6

Paper F – Questions

F1

A 45-year-old male (ideal body weight 80 kg) has been admitted to the ICU with aspiration pneumonitis. He has developed ARDS. He is being mechanically ventilated (SIMV). Ventilator settings are as follows:

F_iO_2	0.8
Tidal volume	760 ml
Respiratory rate	10/min
PEEP	10 cmH$_2$O
Peak airway pressure	40 cmH$_2$O
Plateau airway pressure	37 cmH$_2$O

Blood gas results are:

pH	7.35
P_aO_2	8.5 kPa
P_aCO_2	5.0 kPa
Bicarbonate	24 mmol/l
BE	−0.8
SaO$_2$	90%

What would be the most appropriate next step in this patient's management?
a. Refer for extracorporeal membrane oxygenation (ECMO)
b. Pronate patient
c. Commence intravenous steroids
d. Increase F_iO_2 and/or perform recruitment manoeuvres
e. Reduce tidal volumes and adopt strategy of permissive hypercapnia

---

Practice Single Best Answer Questions for the Final FRCA, ed. Hozefa Ebrahim, Khalid Hasan, Mark Tindall, Michael Clarke and Natish Bindal. Published by Cambridge University Press. © Cambridge University Press 2013.

118

F2

Paravertebral blocks are useful for providing analgesia for a wide range of surgery. They avoid many of the potential difficulties of neuraxial analgesia, but have potential complications of their own.

Which of the following is true?

a. Intrapleural injection of local anaesthetic will result in severe impairment of respiratory function.
b. Pneumothoraces caused during paravertebral blocks are generally small and can be managed conservatively unless the patient is symptomatic.
c. Total spinal block occurs in 4%–5% of cases.
d. Pronounced hypotension is common due to sympathetic block.
e. A urinary catheter is required for any block below T4 in order to prevent urinary retention.

F3

A 54-year-old patient has had a previous spinal fusion for spondylolisthesis. Five years after the fusion, she presents with back pain radiating to her left foot with no effects on motor or excretory function. She has had appropriate conservative management including codeine. After 3 months she requires reoperation. The least useful perioperative pain management adjuvants for this patient would be:

a. Premedication with clonidine and/or gabapentin
b. Incisional local anaesthetic infiltration
c. Intravenous paracetamol
d. Intravenous coxib
e. Intraoperative administration of nitrous oxide

F4

You are called to A&E to see a 35-year-old female with acute asthma. She is confused and exhausted. You perform a rapid sequence induction and intubate with a size 8.0 endotracheal tube, but are finding it impossible to ventilate her and the saturations drop to 75% on 100% oxygen.

What do you do next?

a. Check the position and patency of the endotracheal tube
b. Suspect a tension pneumothorax and attempt a needle decompression
c. Administer further salbutamol and ipratropium nebulizers
d. Commence a magnesium infusion
e. Request an urgent chest X-ray

F5

An 8-month-old infant with a Chiari type II malformation and associated hydrocephalus is listed for revision of a blocked ventriculo-peritoneal shunt. Her parents say that she has been irritable, not feeding well and has vomited once today.

Which of the following drugs would be best avoided during her anaesthetic?

a. Suxamethonium
b. Alfentanil

c. Sevoflurane
d. Nitrous oxide
e. Isoflurane

F6

A significant component of pain experienced after abdominal surgery is related to the abdominal wall incision.

Which of the following abdominal wall nerve blocks would be most suitable following total abdominal hysterectomy via Pfannenstiel incision?
a. Iliohypogastric nerve block
b. Ilioinguinal nerve block
c. Transverse abdominis plane block (bilateral)
d. Rectus sheath block (bilateral)
e. Iliohypogastric and ilioinguinal nerve block

F7

A 76-year-old male is admitted to the cardiac intensive care unit after aortic valve replacement. On the second postoperative day, he is diagnosed to have acute renal failure (ARF).

Which of the following statements regarding the RIFLE classification for ARF is false?
a. R (Risk) – UO <0.5 ml/kg per hour for 6 hours
b. I (Injury) – two-fold increase in serum creatinine, GFR decrease >50%
c. F (Failure) – UO <0.5 ml/kg per hour for 12 hours
d. L (Loss) – complete loss of renal function for > 4 weeks
e. It has been evaluated in cardiac surgical patients

F8

An 85-year-old Afro-Caribbean woman has presented on your trauma list for reduction of a Colles' fracture. She has a history of sickle cell disease and ischaemic heart disease.

Which of the following statements regarding intravenous regional anaesthesia is true?
a. It should be not used in day-case surgery due to the risk of local anaesthetic toxicity
b. It is an appropriate anaesthetic technique for this patient
c. Injection into an ante-cubital fossa vein is preferred
d. Bupivicaine is preferred over prilocaine due to the risk of methaemoglobinaemia
e. At least 20 minutes should pass before the tourniquet is deflated

F9

Scoring systems are commonly used for patients admitted to intensive care. With regard to scoring systems in the critically ill, which of the following is true?
a. The APACHE II (acute physiology and chronic evaluation) maximum score is 80
b. The simplified acute physiology score (SAPS) is a first-day scoring system
c. The mortality prediction model (MPM) is a repetitive scoring system
d. The multiple organ dysfunction score (MODS) scores five organ systems
e. The sepsis-related organ failure assessment (SOFA) scores five organ systems

F10

A 75-year-old male with advanced prostate cancer complains of severe thoracic back pain. An MRI scan reveals localized metastatic bone deposits which do not require surgery. His prognosis is a further 6 months' survival.

Which treatment would be most effective at treating his pain?
a. Bisphosphonates
b. Radiotherapy
c. Oral opioids
d. Intrathecal opioids
e. Intravenous ketamine

F11

You are asked to anaesthetize a 34-year-old lady for insertion of a transjugular intrahepatic porto-systemic shunt. She is suffering from Budd–Chiari syndrome and has large tense ascites. She has no other past medical history and gives no history of reflux. The procedure has been attempted twice under local anaesthesia, but she was unable to tolerate the procedure due to discomfort.

Your anaesthetic plan is to:
a. Ask the physicians and radiologists to attempt the procedure under local anaesthesia again, with larger volumes of local anaesthetic
b. Ask the physicians to improve her respiratory function by draining the ascites first
c. Ask the physicians to perform the procedure again with sedation
d. Provide regional anaesthesia with a cervical plexus block, a large iv access, invasive arterial monitoring and cardiovascular stability, with blood products available
e. Provide general anaesthesia with an ETT, a large iv access, invasive arterial monitoring and cardiovascular stability, with blood products available

F12

Intra-operative cell salvage (ICS) is a technique that allows the blood lost during a surgical procedure to be returned to the patient in an attempt to avoid risks of autologous transfusion. It requires the shed blood to be processed by a machine which filters, washes and centrifuges blood aspirated from the surgical site, to allow only the red cell component to be re-infused.

Which of the following is an absolute contra-indication to the use of cell salvage?
a. Obstetric surgery
b. Surgery involving malignancy
c. Bowel contents in the surgical field
d. Where substances not licensed for iv use (e.g. iodine) are in the operative field
e. Sickle cell trait

F13

You are anaesthetizing a 4-year-old child for unilateral squint correction. The child is breathing spontaneously on sevoflurane. Her heart rate drops to 40 bpm.

The most likely cause is:
a. Traction on medial rectus muscle
b. Oxygen saturation of 92%

c. Her end-tidal carbon dioxide is 7.5 kPa
d. Traction on lateral rectus muscle
e. End-tidal sevoflurane concentration of 3.5%

F14

A 4-month old baby has had diarrhoea and vomiting for the past 3 days. Mum is worried because he has only had one wet nappy in the last 24 hours. His last weight was 8 kg. On examination his heart rate is 160 bpm, he is restless, has a sunken fontanelle and reduced skin turgor.

Which of the following statements is most accurate?
a. The child has approximately 5% dehydration and fluid requirements should be calculated as: deficit 50 ml/kg + maintenance 100 ml/kg per day
b. The child has 10% dehydration and requires initial fluid resuscitation 20 ml/kg and then: deficit 100 ml/kg + maintenance 100 ml/kg per day
c. The child has 10% dehydration and his fluid requirement is: deficit 100 ml/kg + maintenance 100 ml/kg per day
d. The fluid management is administration of sufficient fluids to achieve a urine output of 0.5 ml/kg/per hour
e. The child is severely dehydrated and requires urgent resuscitation of 20 ml/kg followed by: deficit 150 ml/kg + maintenance 100 ml/kg/per day

F15

Spinal cord stimulation is a neuromodulatory technique used in the management of chronic pain.

Which of the following conditions is most likely to respond to spinal cord stimulation?
a. Amputation pain
b. Intercostal neuralgia, e.g. post-thoracotomy
c. Pain associated with spinal cord damage
d. Perineal pain
e. Refractory angina

F16

Laplace's law is relevant to both cardiovascular and respiratory physiology relating wall tension to pressure and radius in fluid-filled systems.

Which of the following represents Laplace's law?
a. wall tension = pressure × wall thickness / radius
b. pressure = radius × wall thickness / wall tension
c. radius × wall tension / thickness = pressure
d. wall tension = pressure × radius / wall thickness
e. wall tension = pressure × wall thickness / radius

F17

You are called to theatre to provide anaesthesia for an emergency Caesarean section on a lady with an umbilical cord prolapse.

Which of the following would be appropriate in this patient's management?
a. Sodium citrate 0.3M (30 ml) will provide sufficient prophylaxis against acid aspiration for the duration of the operation and recovery
b. Induction should be via rapid sequence induction, using thiopental (7.5 mg/kg)
c. Succinylcholine (1 mg/kg) is the neuromuscular blocking agent of choice
d. Cricoid pressure of 20–40 N should be kept in place following induction, until confirmation of tracheal intubation
e. Prophylactic LMWH should be given 4 hours after the end of surgery

F18

Marfan's syndrome is associated with many anatomical features.

Which is not a feature of Marfan's syndrome?
a. Aortic regurgitation
b. Aortic dissection
c. Patent ductus arteriosus
d. Descending thoracic aortic aneurysm
e. Arched palate

F19

With regard to intrathecal opioids, which of the following statements is true?
a. Cephalad movement of opioids injected into the CSF is partly due to expansion and relaxation of the brain, occurring as a result of the cardiac cycle
b. Intrathecal opioids bind receptors in lamina IV of the dorsal horn
c. μ-receptor activation is due to G protein-mediated calcium channel opening
d. Fentanyl has a low volume of distribution within the spinal cord
e. Morphine has limited cephalad spread when injected into the CSF

F20

COPD is associated with respiratory and non-respiratory effects.

Which of the following statements is most accurate?
a. Mucus hypersecretion is due to hypertrophy of goblet cells
b. COPD is associated with chronic bronchitis in fewer than 20% of cases
c. Erythromycin tends to decrease theophylline plasma concentration
d. Hypoxia in COPD patients is due mainly to V/Q mismatch
e. COPD patients with hypoxia and acidosis should be ventilated to normocapnoea

F21

A 58-year-old lady is scheduled to undergo a coronary artery bypass grafting procedure with cardiopulmonary bypass (CPB). In order to minimize the risk of acute kidney injury, which strategy should be avoided intraoperatively?
a. Extra-corporeal leukodepletion
b. Autologous red cell transfusion
c. Haemofiltration during CPB
d. Off-pump coronary artery bypass surgery
e. Moderate haemodilution

F22

Around 40 000 transurethral resection of the prostate (TURP) are performed every year in the UK. Mortality may be as high as 1%. Recognition of acute physiological changes is important in assuring quality of care for patients undergoing TURP.

Which of the following is most accurate?
a. Pain fibres from the prostate originate from the lower part of the lumbar plexus
b. Glycine 2.2% is the most commonly used irrigation fluid in the UK
c. There is evidence to show that spinal anaesthesia has better outcomes than general anaesthesia for TURP
d. Shoulder pain in patients who have had spinal anaesthesia may indicate prostatic capsular rupture
e. Hypotension should be treated by aggressive fluid resuscitation

F23

Carcinoid syndrome results from the secretion of vasoactive and other substances from certain tumours. These have systemic effects relevant to anaesthesia.

Regarding the anaesthetic management of carcinoid syndrome:
a. Patients with asymptomatic carcinoid tumours, or *simple carcinoid disease*, do not need to be managed in the same way as patients with *carcinoid syndrome*
b. Suxamethonium is contra-indicated, as the fasciculations increase intra-abdominal pressure
c. Severe hypotension on induction may be treated with inotropes
d. There is an association with right-sided heart disease, caused by myocardial plaque formation and endocardial fibrosis of the right heart valves
e. A pulmonary artery catheter is indicated

F24

A 78-year-old man with chronic renal impairment, hypertension and peripheral vascular disease presents to the emergency department with abdominal pain. A CT scan shows a leaking, 7-cm juxtarenal aneurysm. He is cross-matched for 6 units of packed red blood cells and 6 units of fresh frozen plasma and given 1000 ml of colloid. The blood products will be in theatre in 10 minutes. In the anaesthetic room, his blood pressure is 95/52, with a heart rate of 88 bpm. The surgeons are scrubbed. An arterial line is *in situ*. The next most appropriate step is:
a. Proceed with a rapid sequence induction, secure the airway, and tell the surgeons to open the abdomen and cross clamp the aorta
b. Site a central venous line under local anaesthetic
c. Increase rate of fluid resuscitation
d. Transfer the patient to theatre, keep him warm, but do not proceed with anaesthesia until the blood products are in theatre
e. Contact the on-call haematologist to request recombinant factor VII

F25

You are asked to sedate a 32-year-old man with severe learning difficulties for an MRI scan of the head. He is uncooperative and impossible to communicate with. There is a carer present who is able to assist.

Which of the following is the most appropriate initial anaesthetic plan to enable the MRI to take place?

a. Secure iv access using necessary restraint and administer iv midazolam in incremental doses
b. Secure iv access using necessary restraint and sedate with propofol iv using a target controlled infusion (TCI)
c. Administer an intramuscular (im) injection of ketamine 10 mg/kg
d. Administer temazepam 30 mg orally on the ward 1 hour before the scan and then conduct an inhalational induction in the MRI suite using sevoflurane
e. Administer temazepam 20 mg orally on the ward one hour before the scan then secure IV access in the MRI suite, followed by propfol TCI sedation

F26

A 16-year-old male attends for an emergency appendicectomy under general anaesthesia. He undergoes a rapid sequence induction with thiopentone and suxamethonium. In recovery he makes no attempt to breathe or cough, he becomes tachycardic and hypertensive, and sweating and pupillary dilatation are evident. Anaesthesia is maintained for 2 hours, at which point he begins to breathe.

Which of the following is this patient's most likely genotype for plasmacholinesterase?

a. Eu : Ea
b. Eu : Eu
c. Ea : Ea
d. Eu : Ef
e. Eu : Es

F27

You are scheduled to anaesthetize a 78-year-old gentleman for an endovascular aortic aneurysm repair (EVAR) in the radiology suite.

Which of the following is the most appropriate statement?

a. The use of a regional technique such as an epidural or CSE is associated with reduced morbidity and mortality
b. A left radial arterial line is usually sited for beat-to-beat monitoring
c. Deployment of the graft in the aorta usually causes some discomfort if a regional anaesthetic technique has been used
d. Bleeding can still occur and the incidence of red cell transfusion is similar to elective open repair
e. Post-operative renal dysfunction is not infrequent

F28

A 65-year-old female is undergoing emergency laparotomy for suspected diverticular perforation. Faeces are seen within the abdominal cavity. The blood pressure has slowly dropped and you have commenced noradrenaline following fluid resuscitation. S_pO_2 is reading 92% and falling, the peak airway pressure is 30 cmH$_2$O having previously been 16 cmH$_2$O. The trachea is shifted to the left. There is decreased chest expansion and a dull percussion note on the left-hand side with reduced air entry also noted on that side.

The most likely diagnosis is:
a. Right-sided tension pneumothorax
b. Right-sided endobronchial intubation
c. Left-sided tension pneumothorax
d. Blocked endotracheal tube
e. Left-sided pleural effusion

F29

A 58-year-old male with COPD is undergoing oesophagectomy. A left-sided double lumen tube is inserted at induction. After 1 hour the S_pO_2 reads 88%. The pulse oximeter is placed correctly and there is a good trace. The patient is receiving F_iO_2 1.0, tidal volume 500 ml, respiratory rate 10, PEEP 5 cmH$_2$O.

What is your first action?
a. Increase tidal volume to 600 ml
b. Clamp the pulmonary artery to the non-dependent lung
c. Check tube position with a fibre-optic bronchoscope
d. Inform surgeon and re-inflate collapsed lung
e. Add CPAP 5 cmH$_2$O to upper lung

F30

A 63-year-old man presents for arthrodesis of his ankle under general anaesthesia. His has a history of heart failure, well-controlled hypertension and ischaemic heart disease. He underwent balloon angioplasty 9 months ago. He can now walk half a mile at his own pace without getting short of breath or angina. He takes aspirin, clopidogrel, bisoprolol, ramipril, simvastatin and bendroflumethiazide. On arrival in the anaesthetic room, the ward nurse tells you he has not had any of his medication that day, but had all of his drugs yesterday. The most appropriate next step is:
a. Cancel surgery and reschedule for another day
b. Site an arterial line, draw up vasopressors and proceed with general anaesthesia
c. Convert to a regional technique
d. Return the patient to the ward to take his medication and reschedule surgery for later on the list
e. Continue with general anaesthesia, but give iv beta-blocker at induction

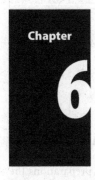

Chapter

6

Paper F – Answers

F1

Answer: e.

This patient has ARDS and has refractory hypoxaemia. They have a P/F ratio <26.6. Arterial oxygen saturations above 88% are acceptable. In order to achieve these results, however the patient is being over-ventilated with excessive tidal volumes. According to ARDSnet ventilatory strategies, a tidal volume of 6 ml/kg ideal body weight should be aimed for. The patient's plateau airway pressures are excessive. In this instance the ventilatory strategy has to be amended to a 'lung protective' strategy in which tidal volume will be reduced in line with ARDSnet and, should this result in hypercapnia, then this will be tolerated.

Should the patient become more hypoxic and need increasing F_iO_2 following this change in ventilation, then further options include optimizing PEEP, pronation and consideration for specialist care such as high frequency oscillatory ventilation (HFOV) and extra-corporal membrane oxygenation (ECMO).

Winter, B. The refractory hypoxaemia guidelines. *J Intens Care Soc* 2011; **12** (1): 8

F2

Answer: b.

Paravertebral blocks were described in the early twentieth century. Their use declined until the early 1980s, when they were brought back into the mainstream. A series of publications since then have established them as a useful technique with a favourable side effect profile.

The major issues with paravertebral blocks are failure of the block (in around 5%–10% of cases), haematoma and pneumothorax. Pneumothoraces are indeed generally minor and can often be managed conservatively. If they are large or cause respiratory embarrassment, it may be necessary to insert an intercostal drain and patients should be warned about this as part of their consent. Intrapleural injection of local anaesthetic is used by some as a deliberate method of providing analgesia. If intrapleural needle placement is detected, a decision can be made whether to proceed with deliberate injection of local anaesthetic or to withdraw the needle and retry at a lower or higher level. Total spinal block is exceedingly rare, being reported twice in the worldwide literature. Urinary retention does not occur with paravertebral blocks alone and a catheter is not required for this reason.

Practice Single Best Answer Questions for the Final FRCA, ed. Hozefa Ebrahim, Khalid Hasan, Mark Tindall, Michael Clarke and Natish Bindal. Published by Cambridge University Press. © Cambridge University Press 2013.

Tighe SQM, Greene MD, Rajadurai N. Paravertebral block. *Contin Educ Anaesth Crit Care Pain* 2010; **10**(5): 133–137

F3

Answer: e.

Both the α_2-agonists and anticonvulsants are useful adjuvants in opioid tolerance. Local anaesthetic infiltration in this case covers the skin sensation for 6–8 hours. Intravenous paracetamol and a COX_2-inhibitor should be maintained until the oral preparations the patient has used previously can be recommenced. While nitrous oxide is an NMDA antagonist, the effect of the drug is transient and will have the least effect on postoperative pain.

Rosenquist RW, Rosenberg J. Postoperative Pain Guidelines. *Reg Anesth Pain Med* 2003; **28**: 279–288

F4

Answer: a.

This question is really more about testing your ability to apply common sense in a stressful situation, rather than the management of acute severe asthma. If it is impossible to bag a patient after intubation, it is essential you ensure patency and position of your endotracheal tube. Severe bronchospasm may make ventilation very difficult, and only very low tidal volumes may be achievable, but complete obstruction to any gas flow is unlikely. If the patient is truly impossible to ventilate, you should disconnect the circuit and manually decompress the chest before further attempts at ventilation.

Once correct placement and patency of the ETT is confirmed, further treatment measures can be instigated. These may include:

- β_2-agonists (nebulized better than iv)
- Anticholinergics
- Steroids
- Magnesium
- Aminophylline
- Ketamine
- Adrenaline
- Volatile anaesthetic agents
- Helium
- ECMO

Gas trapping makes over-distension a hazard and there is a high risk of barotraumas and pneumothoracies. Generally, ventilation strategies should include low tidal volumes and a low respiratory rate with prolonged expiratory times. The use of PEEP is controversial.

Stanley D, Tunnicliffe W. Management of life threatening asthma in adults. *Contin Educ Anaesth Crit Care Pain* 2008; **8**(3): 95–99

F5

Answer: d.

Preoperative assessment in this case should focus on signs and symptoms of raised intracranial pressure (ICP) such as irritability, poor feeding, bulbar symptoms and sleep disturbances. Conscious level using an age-specific Glasgow Coma Scale (GCS) should be ascertained.

Anaesthetic induction should aim to avoid hypercapnia, hypoxia, variations in blood pressure and increases in cerebral blood flow (CBF) that may cause further rises in ICP. An iv induction with propofol or thiopental and neuromuscular block is therefore ideal. Ketamine causes an increase in ICP and is not recommended. If a rapid sequence induction is necessary, the small increase in ICP associated with the use of suxamethonium can be attenuated by the use of opioids or pre-curization doses of non-depolarizing neuromuscular blocking agents. Opioids such as remifentanil or alfentanil should be used to attenuate the hypertensive responses to laryngoscopy, intubation and surgery.

If the child is distressed or has difficult iv access, a smooth gas induction may be better than the raised ICP associated with crying or struggling. Sevoflurane confers benefits over other volatile agents (e.g. isoflurane), in this situation. Its odour is well tolerated and the likelihood of airway irritation, laryngospasm and breath holding are reduced. There is also greater haemodynamic stability and rapid emergence after prolonged surgery with sevoflurane compared with isoflurane. At concentrations <1 minimum alveolar concentration (MAC), there is no associated increase in CBF.

Nitrous oxide is best avoided in neurosurgery as it causes significant increases in CBF and cerebral metabolic oxygen requirement ($CMRO_2$). It may also trigger postoperative nausea and vomiting with subsequent rises in ICP. The volume of gas-filled spaces may also increase with the potential for expansion of pneumocephalus and raised ICP postoperatively.

Furay C, Howell T. Paediatric neuroanaesthesia. *Contin Educ Anaesth Crit Care Pain* 2010; 10(6): 172–176

F6

Answer: c.

A Pfannenstiel incision is usually made 1–2 fingerbreadths above the pubic crest with a length of 10–14 cm. This corresponds to the L1 dermatome. The rectus sheath block is used for analgesia after umbilical or incisional hernia repairs and other midline surgical incisions. Ilioinguinal and iliohypogastric nerve blocks can provide good analgesia for most operations in the inguinal region, however, need to be performed in tandem and bilaterally if the incision crosses the midline.

The aim of the TAP block is to block the sensory nerves of the anterior abdominal wall before they pierce the musculature to innervate the abdomen. The block can be performed either by using a landmark technique or with the aid of ultrasound. The aim is to place a large volume of local anaesthetic in the fascial plane between the internal oblique and transversus abdominis which contains the nerves from T7 to L1. The onset of the sensory block appears to be relatively slow, taking up to 60 min to reach maximal effect. Ideally the block is placed at the start of surgery to give adequate time for the onset of sensory analgesia. For incisions at or crossing the midline, bilateral TAP blocks are indicated.

The TAP block provides analgesia for the abdominal wall but not for the visceral contents and is ideally used as part of a multimodal approach to analgesia. Good postoperative analgesia and a decrease in morphine requirements for up to 48 h after operation have been demonstrated after a variety of abdominal surgeries. Used bilaterally, it may be a simple alternative in patients for whom an epidural is not possible, although there is no comparative data as to the relative effectiveness of the two techniques.

Yarwood J, Berrill A. Nerve blocks of the anterior abdominal wall. *Contin Educ Anaesth Crit Care Pain* 2010; **10**(6): 182–186

F7
Answer: c.

Acute renal failure is defined as a decrease in the function of the kidney, which occurs very rapidly. It can vary from a mild renal impairment of function to a serious irreversible condition needing replacement therapy. The RIFLE classification was published in 2004 and has three levels of severity (R, risk; I, injury; F, failure) and two outcomes (L, loss; E, end-stage). These RIFLE criteria were created by the Acute Dialysis Quality Initiative based on assessment of patients in intensive care and cardiac surgery.

- R (risk) – serum creatinine increase 1.5-fold, GFR decrease >25%, UO <0.5 ml/kg per hour for 6 hours
- I (injury) – serum creatinine increase two-fold, GFR decrease >50%, UO <0.5 ml/kg per hour for 12 hours
- F (failure) – serum creatinine increase three-fold, GFR decrease >75% or serum creatinine >350 μmol/l with increase >44 μmol/l, UO <0.3 ml/kg per hour for 24 hours or anuria for 12 hours
- L (loss) – complete loss of renal function for > 4 weeks
- E (end-stage) – complete loss of renal function for > 3 months

Webb ST, Allen JSD. Perioperative renal protection. *Contin Educ Anaesth Crit Care Pain* 2008; **8**(5): 176–180

F8
Answer: e.

The Bier block was first described in 1908. The patient should be starved and monitored as for any procedure. Intravenous cannulae are placed in each hand and the limb is exsanguinated. A double cuff tourniquet is applied to the upper arm and the proximal cuff is inflated to twice the systolic blood pressure. Five to ten minutes after slow injection of the local anaesthetic, the distal cuff may be inflated and the proximal cuff deflated to reduce tourniquet-related pain. The tourniquet must remain inflated for at least 20 minutes.

Prilocaine 0.5% is the safest local anaesthetic to use. For the average-sized patient, 40 ml should be adequate. Lignocaine without adrenaline may also be used, but bupivacaine is avoided because of its toxicity, particularly to the myocardium. The major complications from the procedure arise from local anaesthetic toxicity when the tourniquet is deflated too soon. Intravenous regional anaesthesia is not appropriate for a patient with sickle cell disease due to the risk of tissue ischaemia.

Yentis SM, Hirsch NP, Smith GB. *Anaesthesia and Intensive Care A–Z: An Encyclopedia of Principles and Practice*, 3rd edn, 2012 London, UK: Butterworth-Heinemann

F9

Answer: b.

Scoring systems are commonly used for patients admitted to intensive care. They quantify illness severity and the likelihood of in-hospital mortality. They are of use as an audit tool and can allow individual units to compare their performance over time.

The variables in a scoring system can be grouped into five categories: age, co-morbidities, physiological abnormalities, acute diagnosis and interventions.

Methods used for scoring systems include:

- *Anatomical scoring* – mainly used in trauma and depend on the anatomical area involved such as the injury severity score (ISS)
- *Therapeutic weighted scores* – based on the assumption that the more severe the illness is, the more frequent and complex the interventions will be, such as the therapeutic intervention scoring system (TISS)
- *Organ-specific scoring* – based on the assumption that the more severe the illness is, the more organ systems will be involved (SOFA)
- *Physiological assessment* – based on the degree of derangement of physiological variables (APACHE, SAPS)
- *Simple scales* – based on clinical judgement
- *Disease specific* – e.g. Ranson's criteria for acute pancreatitis

Scoring systems are usually designed to be applied on the first day of critical admission but can be repetitive with data collected throughout the critical care admission. Types of scoring system are shown below:

- *First-day scoring systems* – APACHE, SAPS, MPM;
- *Repetitive scoring systems* – SOFA, MODS.

The APACHE II maximum score is 71. A score of 25 represents a predicted mortality of 50% and a score over 35 represents a predicted mortality of 80%. APACHE II remains the mostly widely used severity scoring system. The MODS scores six organ systems and the SOFA also scores six organ systems.

Bouch CD, Thompson JP. Severity scoring systems in the critically ill. *Contin Educ Anaesth Crit Care Pain* 2008; 8(5): 181–185

F10

Answer: b.

Though metastatic bone disease commonly causes pain, this can be of variable severity and up to 25% of cases can be pain free. Metastatic bone pain is usually a worsening dull continuous ache which can be exacerbated by movement. The mechanisms of pain from bony deposits include soft tissue damage, inflammation, nerve compression and infiltration, pathological fractures and collapse. Pharmacological treatment of cancer pain should always invoke the WHO analgesic ladder, comprising paracetamol, weak then strong opioids and adjuvants as severity increases. However, radiotherapy is the single most effective intervention for metastatic bone pain with 70% of patients obtaining significant pain relief and a complete response in one-third. Bisphosphonates are potent inhibitors of osteolysis and bone resorption and have been shown to alleviate bony pain but are not first-line treatments. Good-quality trials looking at the efficacy of intrathecal or epidural opioids for cancer pain are lacking so these remain unproven, though they have been used successfully for refractory neuropathic cancer pain. Ketamine has been used for refractory cancer pain as an adjuvant to opioids, though again good-quality evidence to support its use is not yet available.

Janes R, Saart T. Oncologic therapy in cancer pain, in Stannard C, Kalso E, Ballantyne J. *Evidence-based Chronic Pain, Management*, 1st edn, 2010. Wiley-VCH, 311–336

Oxberry SG, Simpson KH. Pharmacotherapy for cancer pain. *Contin Educ Anaesth Crit Care Pain* 2005;5(6):203–206

F11

Answer: e.

It is unlikely that they will succeed with local anaesthesia if they have tried twice before and it is unfair to the patient if she finds it distressing or uncomfortable. The question states the procedure was terminated twice due to discomfort, not hypoxia. However, this does have to be borne in mind for people with large, tense ascites. Sedation is an option, but the potential for the respiratory depressant effects of sedation on patients with liver disease with pulmonary dysfunction (from ascites or porto-pulmonary associations), as well as their prolonged action of sedative drugs, the risk of aspiration, the risk of precipitating encephalopathy and a prolonged procedure make a general anaesthetic with a *secure* airway the treatment of choice.

Steadman R. Anaesthesia for liver transplant surgery. *Anesthesiol Clin N Am* 2004; **22**: 687–711

Morgan GE, Mikhail MS. *Clinical Anesthesiolgy*, 4th edn, USA: McGraw-Hill, 797–801

F12

Answer: c.

a. and b. were previously contra-indications to ICS because of concerns about amniotic fluid embolism or dissemination of malignancy. The use of leukocyte depletion filters makes ICS a practical technique in these conditions.
c. The use of ICS in the presence of bowel contents is contra-indicated unless there is catastrophic haemorrhage.
d. Provided the ICS suction is temporarily stopped, the surgical field irrigated with saline and cleared with normal theatre suction, ICS can be continued.
e. There are concerns relating to the use of ICS in sickle cell *disease*, although the decision to use ICS should be made on a patient-by-patient basis.

UK Cell Salvage Action Group. *Intraoperative Cell Salvage Education Workbook*. http://www.transfusionguidelines.org.uk/docs/pdfs/bbt-03_icsag_workbook-0812_all.pdf Accessed 20/02/12

F13

Answer: a.

The child presenting for squint surgery may be otherwise fit and well or may have associated diseases such as cerebral palsy, hydrocephalus, myopathies or other chromosomal abnormalities. Attention should be paid to these at the preoperative visit.

It is well known that strabismus surgery is associated with oculocardiac reflex. This is a bradycardic response to traction on any of the extraocular eye muscles (more commonly the medial rectus), which may also result in sinus arrest or major dysrhythmias. Afferent pathways are via the occipital branch of the trigeminal nerve and the efferent is via the vagus. Oculocardiac reflex occurs in approximately 60% of children undergoing squint surgery. On removal of traction the bradycardia resolves almost instantaneously. Prevention will involve administering atropine 20 mcg/kg, which may be given at induction as a routine or following a reflex event in theatre.

Most cases are anaesthetized with the child spontaneously breathing, but it should be noted that light anaesthesia or hypercarbia increases the risk of oculocardiac reflex.

Strabismus surgery is associated with significant postoperative nausea and vomiting (PONV), which may be linked to oculocardiac reflex, since children who have bradycardias intraoperatively are at increased risk of PONV. Multi-modal antiemetic prophylaxis should be administered.

The incidence of malignant hyperthermia is increased in patients with squint (still rare), but vigilance should be high.

James I. Anaesthesia for paediatric eye surgery. *Contin Educ Anaesth Crit Care Pain* 2008; **8** (1): 5–10

F14

Answer: c.

This child has clinical signs of dehydration in keeping with a deficit of approximately 10%. A mildly dehydrated child (5%) has signs of thirst and may be restless, but has normal skin turgor, heart rate, fontanelle and moist mucous membranes. Greater than 10% dehydration will have evidence of shock and require volume resuscitation in the form of 20 ml/kg boluses.

The deficit fluid replacement can be estimated by the degree of dehydration. For example, 10% dehydration means the child has lost 10 ml per 100 g of weight (100 ml/kg). They will therefore require this to be added to their maintenance over the following 24 hours.

The daily maintenance requirement can be calculated by

- 100 ml/kg for 0–10 kg
- 50 ml/kg for subsequent 10 kg
- 20 ml/kg for subsequent kg

For example, this 8-kg boy would require maintenance of $100 \times 8 = 800$ ml over 24 hours = 33 ml/hr. A 22 kg child would require $1000 + 500 + 40 = 1540$ ml over 24 hours = 64 ml/h.

This child's overall fluid requirement for the following 24 hours is: deficit (100 ml $\times$ 8 kg = 800 ml) + maintenance (100 ml $\times$ 8 kg = 800 ml) = 1600 ml/24 hours = 67 ml/h.

In adults a urine output of 0.5 ml/kg is generally acceptable; however, in infants the target should be > 2 ml/kg and for children it is > 1 ml/kg

If this child required surgery for any reason, the dehydration should ideally be corrected preoperatively. A healthy child coming for elective surgery will have a fluid deficit of the number of hours starvation multiplied by the hourly maintenance requirement. As a guide, approximately 50% of this can be replaced over the first hour and the remainder over the subsequent 2 hours.

Cunliffe M. Fluid and electrolyte management in children. *Contin Educ Anaesth Crit Care Pain* 2003; 3(1): 1–4

Samuels M, Wieteska S (eds). Appendix B: Fluid and Electrolyte Management, in *Advanced Paediatric Life Support, The Practical Approach*. 5th edn. 2011. London: Wiley-Blackwell, 279–289

F15

Answer: e.

Spinal cord stimulation (SCS) is a neuromodulatory technique that is becoming increasingly popular in the management of chronic pain. There is increasing evidence for its role in the management of neuropathic pain, CRPS, refractory angina and ischaemic pain associated with peripheral vascular disease.

A spinal cord stimulator is an implantable system that delivers electrical impulses via leads to large diameter afferents in the dorsal columns. These afferents inhibit pain transmission rostrally and the patient feels paraesthesia over the area the pain was felt. Neurotransmitters involved in this neuromodulation include gamma amino-butyric acid (GABA), which may in turn inhibit excitatory neurotransmitters such as aspartate and glutamate.

The leads that allow SCS are sited percutaneously via a modified Tuohy needle and are then directed to an appropriate level under fluoroscopic guidance. Initially, an external pulse generator is used to trial the SCS for a number of days to assess efficacy before the patient returns to theatre to have an implantable pulse generator sited; this is about the size of a cardiac pacemaker.

The more frequent complications associated with SCS are technical problems such as lead migration and lead fracture rather than post-surgical complications such as infection or CSF leak.

Raphael JH, Mutagi HS, Kapur S. Spinal cord stimulation and its anaesthetic implications. *Cont Educ Anaesth Crit Care Pain* 2009; 9(3): 78–81

F16

Answer: d.

Increases in both pressure and radius increase wall tension. b. and c. can be re-arranged to make wall tension the subject of the equation, showing that they are both incorrect.

In cardiovascular physiology dilated cardiomyopathies are an example of Laplace's law at work. Dilation of the cardiac ventricles increases the tension necessary to provide pressure for forward flow. This, in turn increases myocardial oxygen demand.

Right ventricular failure can occur with relatively small changes in pulmonary afterload due to the compliant nature of the right ventricle. Right ventricular failure can occur in this situation because of increased wall tension and decreased blood supply.

In addition, Laplace's law shows that increasing blood pressure has an effect on the diameter of blood vessels through which blood flows. Increasing the diameter of blood vessels at the same time as increasing the driving pressure can give rise to large increases in blood flow.

In pulmonary physiology Laplace's law explains the lower inflection point on the pressure–volume curve of lung inflation and is part of the rational for the application of CPAP in patients with respiratory embarrassment or PEEP in ventilated patients. At low alveolar volumes, high pressures are required to produce sufficient wall tension to open the pulmonary alveoli. As the size of the alveoli increases, the pressure required to produce increases in wall tension rapidly reduces. Applying PEEP reduces the tendency of alveoli to collapse to very small sizes meaning that lower inspiratory pressures are required to give useful tidal volumes.

Adams J, Charlton P. Anaesthesia for microvascular free tissue transfer. *Contin Educ Anaesth Crit Care Pain* 2003; 3(2): 33–37

Kevin LG, Barnard M. Right ventricular failure. *Contin Educ Anaesth Crit Care Pain* 2007; 7 (3): 89–94

Scott T, Swanevelder J. Perioperative myocardial protection. *Contin Educ Anaesth Crit Care Pain* 2009; 9(3): 97–101

F17

Answer: d.

Sodium citrate 0.3M (30 ml) does provide a near instantaneous antacid effect; however, its effects are short-lived, and it may have worn off by the time of emergence. Furthermore, its use is to reduce the incidence of pneumonitis following aspiration, and not to prevent aspiration itself. Thiopental is given at a dose of 5 mg/kg. Succinylcholine is given at a dose of 1.5 mg/kg, but higher doses may be required due to increased volume of distribution and relative resistance. Cricoid pressure of 10 N should be applied prior to loss of consciousness, and then increased to 20–40 N following induction. As no central neuraxial blockade has been used, LMWH may be given sooner after surgery.

McGlennan A, Mustafa A. General anaesthesia for Caesarean section. *Contin Educ Anaesth Crit Care Pain* 2009; 9(5): 139–143

F18

Answer: c.

Marfan's syndrome is associated with numerous aortopathies but not patent ductus arteriosus.

Judge DP, Dietz HC. Marfan's syndrome. *Lancet* 2005; 366(9501): 1965–1976

F19

Answer: a.

Intrathecal opioids bind to receptors in laminae I and II of the dorsal horn. Receptor activation leads to G-protein-mediated potassium channel opening in mu and delta receptors and calcium channel closing in kappa receptors. Fentanyl has a high volume of distribution within the CSF due to its high octanol:water partition coefficient. After fentanyl administration, CSF concentrations decrease rapidly and there is limited cephalad spread. Morphine is more hydrophilic than fentanyl with a low octanol:water coefficient. It has a low volume of distribution within the CSF and more readily spreads in a cephalad direction.

Hindle A. Intrathecal opioids in the management of acute postoperative pain. *Contin Educ Anaesth Crit Care Pain* 2008; **8**(3): 81–85

F20

Answer: d.

COPD is a complex disorder in which the pathology includes inflammation of the epithelial lining of the airways, oedema, hypertrophy of mucus secreting glands and an increase in the number of goblet cells. The goblet cells themselves are of normal structure and size.

Chronic bronchitis is often considered one of the major forms of COPD, the other being emphysema. Patients can be broadly categorized into the two categories classically represented by blue bloaters (chronic bronchitis) and pink puffers (emphysema), but it is important to realize that there is cross-over in the pathologies and that some patients do not fit neatly into either group.

Theophylline is a difficult drug to manage, particularly in patients who are often taking a number of other medications for a range of other diseases. It has a narrow therapeutic range and plasma concentration can be increased or decreased by drugs or diseases. Erythromycin tends to increase plasma theophylline concentration.

COPD patients often survive with lower than expected oxygen tensions. They also tend to be hypercapnic, but renally compensated. Ventilating these patients to normocapneoa makes them alkalotic with all its attendant issues. Improper ventilation tends to increase time of ventilation and is associated with poor outcomes.

Hogg JC, Chu F, Utokaparch S *et al.* The nature of small-airway obstruction in chronic obstructive pulmonary disease. *NEJM* 2004; **350**(26): 2645–2653

F21

Answer: b.

Four per cent of the patients undergoing cardiac surgery with cardiopulmonary bypass (CPB) develop acute kidney injury needing dialysis. This may be due to the production of free haemoglobin, which can in turn increase free iron in renal tubular cells, impairing its function. Removal of polymorphonuclear cells by using an effective filter during CPB may actually improve the renal and pulmonary functions of these patients. Although off-pump coronary artery bypass graft (CABG) preserves kidney function to a greater degree, it is not suitable in patients with severe coronary artery disease, as severe haemodynamic changes occur when the heart is manipulated. Haemodilution decreases the haematocrit of blood and hence its viscosity, ultimately improving the rheology of renal blood flow and protecting the kidney function. This is offset by the fact that dilute blood will have a lower oxygen-carrying capacity, hence severe haemodilution below a haematocrit of 21% must be avoided. Moderate haemodilution to a haematocrit of, 21%–25% has been shown to be most beneficial to the kidneys. Transfusion of RBCs not only increases the haemtocrit and viscosity of blood, but also interacts with CPB to cause severe kidney injury and TRALI.

Webb ST, Allen JSD. Perioperative renal protection. *Contin Educ Anaesth Crit Care Pain* 2008; **8**(5): 176–180
Karkouti K, Beattie WS, Wijeysundera DN, *et al.* Haemodilution during cardiopulmonary bypass is an independent risk factor for acute renal failure in adult cardiac surgery. *J Thorac Cardiovasc Surg* 2005;**129**: 391–400

F22

Answer: d.

Nerves to the prostate arise in the prostatic plexus, which originates in the inferior hypogastric plexus. The prostatic plexus includes sympathetic fibres from T11 to L2 and parasympathetic fibres from S2 to S4. Bladder distension is signalled by the parasympathetic fibres and bladder pain is signalled in sympathetic fibres.

The ideal surgical irrigation fluid is transparent, electrically non-conductive, isotonic and non-toxic. Glycine 1.5% is commonly used in the UK, but has an osmolarity of 220 mosm/l. Other solutions include 3.5% sorbitol and 5% mannitol.

There is very little evidence to show that spinal anaesthesia is better than general, but spinal remains the anaesthetic of choice in the UK. In particular, spinal anaesthesia has the potential advantage of the anaesthetist being able to observe for altered consciousness or fits, which might occur as a result of TUR syndrome. Spinal anaesthesia also offers postoperative analgesia, which may be useful in patients with respiratory compromise. Awake patients complaining of shoulder tip pain may have suffered prostatic capsular rupture.

Severe hypotension during TUR is rare as the legs are elevated, which serves to offset the pooling of blood caused by sympathetic blockade. Hypotension is best treated by judicious use of vasopressors as significant fluid may be absorbed from the surgical irrigation.

Hahn RG. Fluid absorption in endoscopic surgery. *Br J Anaesth* 2006; **96**:8–20
O'Donnell AM, Foo ITH. Anaesthesia for transurethral resection of the prostate. *Contin Educ Anaesth Crit Care Pain* 2009; **9**(3): 92–96

F23

Answer: d.

The risk from suxamethonium is more theoretical than practical. Severe hypotension is best treated with octreotide (10–20 mcg) boluses, as catecholamines will not be effective in an α-or β-blocked patient, and they may trigger kallikrein activation. A pulmonary catheter is only indicated if cardiac complications are evident. Statement a is irrelevant to the question, although the statement is true. The question states 'regarding the anaesthetic management of *carcinoid syndrome*', not carcinoid disease.

Powell B, Mukhtar A, Mills G. Carcinoid: the disease and its implications for anaesthesia. *Contin Educ Anaesth Crit Care Pain* 2011; **11**(1): 9–13

F24

Answer: d.

A leaking aneurysm is a surgical emergency requiring immediate attention. This patient appears to be relatively haemodynamically stable. He has an acceptable blood pressure after minimal fluid resuscitation, is not tachycardic and has been judged stable enough to undergo CT. It is important not to over-resuscitate a leaking aneurysm. A high MAP may dislodge a newly formed thrombus, and haemodilution will reduce the efficacy of the clotting system.

A CVP line is essential, but can be sited once the patient is anaesthetized. Siting it in the anaesthetic room, even with local anaesthesia, can be uncomfortable, and increase the stress response.

Blood leaking into the abdomen can have the effect of tamponading the leak. Opening the abdomen and relieving the tamponade, in conjunction with general anaesthesia, may cause cardiovascular collapse. In this situation, it would be prudent to wait a few minutes for fully cross-matched blood to be available in theatre, so that the haemodynamic instability associated with the start of anaesthesia and surgery can be treated immediately with appropriate volume replacement.

Leonard A, Thompson J. Anaesthesia for ruptured abdominal aortic aneurysm. *Contin Educ Anaesth Crit Care Pain* 2008; **8**: 11–15

F25

Answer: d.

This case highlights a number of challenges for the anaesthetist:

- An uncooperative patient with no insight or capacity to understand any planned intervention
- An environment remote to theatre with staff who may be unfamiliar with the practice of anaesthesia and sedation
- A patient who may have complex co-existing disease
- Anaesthesia in a powerful magnetic field with its associated risks for the patients and staff
- Limited access to the patient during the procedure

Before undertaking the case, a consultant anaesthetist and trained anaesthetic assistant should be present. A full history and examination relevant to anaesthesia should be undertaken. All anaesthetic equipment and monitoring must be MRI compatible.

General anaesthesia is preferred to sedation in this case for a number of reasons. It is imperative that the patient lies still for the entire procedure to ensure that the images obtained are of satisfactory quality. In order to achieve this using sedation, in this patient, it is likely that large doses will be required, which may compromise the airway and/or breathing. The airway is not easily accessible in the scanner. An MRI of the head is likely to take 15–20 minutes.

It will be difficult to restrain an adult patient without the risk of injury to either the patient or staff, so this is not appropriate. Oral premedication should be tried first, followed by induction of general anaesthesia if not contra-indicated. If the patient will not accept oral sedation then intramuscular ketamine is another option in a dose of 10 mg/kg. This acts rapidly to induce a dissociative state of anaesthesia. Minimum monitoring for general anaesthesia must be used and the patient must be recovered to the same standard as with any other procedure under general anaesthetic.

Royal College of Anaesthetists. *Guidance on Provision of Anaesthetic Care in the Non-theatre environment*. Revised 2011

F26
Answer: c.

This patient is likely to have a diagnosis of *suxamethonium apnoea*. Suxamethonium apnoea is an inherited or acquired condition leading to the prolongation of the effect of suxamethonium. The acquired form results from reduced plasma cholinesterase activity, secondary to a number of conditions including pregnancy, renal failure, liver disease, cardiac failure, hypothyroidism, cardiopulmonary bypass, carcinoma and drugs. Acquired suxamethonium apnoea commonly presents with a mild to moderate prolongation of paralysis.

Inherited suxamethonium apnoea is caused by an abnormal gene for plasma cholinesterase on chromosome 6. There are four alleles for plasma cholinesterase:

- Usual (Eu)
- Atypical (Ea)
- Silent (Es)
- Fluoride-resistant (Ef)

Combinations of these alleles lead to ten possible genotypes, of which the most common is Eu : Eu. This occurs in 96% of the Caucasian population and results in normal plasma cholinesterase activity. Heterozygotes for abnormal alleles (e.g. Eu : Ea, Eu : Es, Eu : Ef) are less common and present with moderately prolonged recovery times of up to 30 minutes. The incidence of the homozygous state for the atypical allele (Ea : Ea) is approximately 1:2800 and this leads to a significantly prolonged recovery time of 2 hours. This is most likely in the patient in question. Homozygous forms of the Es and Ef alleles are extremely rare.

The management of suxamethonium apnoea is supportive, comprising maintenance of anaesthesia and ventilation and continuous neuromuscular monitoring until train-of-four (TOF) stimulation elicits four strong twitches. Follow-up care should include an explanation to the patient and plasma cholinesterase assay of the patient and their direct family. Percentage inhibition of cholinesterase by dibucaine can be used to determine the likely genotype: the lower the dibucaine number, the more abnormal the genotype.

Peck TE, Hill SA, Williams M. *Pharmacology for Anaesthesia and Intensive Care*, 2nd edn, 2003. London: Greenwich Medical Media

F27
Answer: e.

EVAR is an increasingly popular procedure, which is often undertaken in a remote site. It has proven advantages of decreased mortality and reduced hospital stay, avoiding all of the inherent complications of an open laparotomy. The patient must be assessed in exactly the same manner as an open repair, focusing in particular on concurrent cardiovascular, respiratory and renal disease. A contingency plan for emergency conversion to open repair must be in place and well rehearsed.

The procedure can be performed under GA, regional anaesthetic or local infiltration, but there is no evidence to support improved outcome with any technique in particular. A right radial arterial line is usually inserted, as rarely the left axillary artery is required for access to the aorta. The deployment of the graft is usually painless.

Bleeding can still occur throughout, particularly from the femoral access incisions, but studies have shown that overall blood loss is in the region of 60% lower compared with open repair.

Copious amounts of radiocontrast elements are used, which may cause renal impairment. The urine output must be monitored and an adequate hydration status maintained. Depending on local guidelines, N-acetylcysteine may be given preoperatively if a degree of renal impairment is already present.

Nataraj V, Mortimer A. *Contin Educ Anaesth Crit Care Pain* 2004; 4(3): 91–94

F28
Answer: b.

This patient has an endobronchial intubation that has resulted in left-sided collapse. Signs of left-sided collapse are tracheal deviation towards the affected side, reduced chest expansion, dull percussion note and reduced breath sounds all on the affected side (left in this case).

During anaesthesia it is possible that the patient may desaturate and airway pressures may increase. The degree to which this occurs is multi-factorial and varies between patients depending on the clinical state.

This is not a typical presentation of a tension pneumothorax. The trachea would move away from the affected side and there would be a hyper-resonant percussion note on the affected side. Airway pressures may increase and the patient would be expected to desaturate. A more precipitous fall in blood pressure would be expected.

Left-sided pleural effusion is incorrect and would not present in this way unless massive. It would have been detected earlier and the trachea would be deviated away from the affected side.

Paramasivan E, Bodenham A. Airleaks, pneumothorax and chest drains. *Contin Educ Anaesth Crit Care Pain* 2008; 8(6): 204–209

F29
Answer: c.

The most common cause for desaturation during the procedure is the accumulation of secretions or migration of the endotracheal tube. A fibre-optic scope should be kept available for use in order to check the tube position in the event of any change in the patient's oxygenation.

If the patient fails to improve after clearance of secretions and the tube is optimally positioned, then the ventilator settings should be reviewed. The F_iO_2 should be increased if the patient isn't receiving F_iO_2 1.0 and CPAP can be administered to the upper lung after informing the surgeon that the lung may partially re-inflate. PEEP can be added to the dependent lung as a further means of improving oxygenation. Further rescue techniques include re-inflating the upper lung and clamping the pulmonary artery to the non-dependent lung.

Eastwood J, Mahajan R. One lung anaesthesia. *Contin Educ Anaesth Crit Care Pain* 2002; 2(3): 83–87

F30

Answer: d.

Dual antiplatelet therapy precludes a regional technique. A combination of general anaesthesia and acute iv beta blockade could result in profound cardiovascular suppression. The POISE study has shown that patients who take beta-blockers should have them continued throughout the perioperative period to reduce cardiovascular morbidity and mortality; however, they should not be started *de novo* due to the risk of acute stroke and an increase in all-cause mortality. It would be unfair and unnecessary to cancel the patient, so option d. is the most appropriate of these actions.

Sear JW, Giles JW, Howard-Alpe G, Foëx P. Perioperative beta-blockade: what does POISE tell us, and was our earlier caution justified? *Br J Anaesth* 2008; 101: 135–138

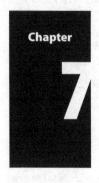

Paper G – Questions

G1

A 61-year-old gentleman attends the anaesthetic preoperative clinic. He is due to attend for a total knee replacement in 6 weeks' time. His past medical history includes a mechanical mitral valve replacement 5 years previously and he is on warfarin. It is decided to discontinue his warfarin 5 days preoperatively.

Select the anticoagulation strategy most appropriate for this patient in the 5 days before surgery:
a. Leave the patient off all anticoagulants because of the high bleeding risk.
b. Give therapeutic dose subcutaneous low molecular weight heparin daily, administering the last dose 24 hours before surgery.
c. Give therapeutic dose subcutaneous low molecular weight heparin daily, with the last dose 12 hours before surgery.
d. Give continuous intravenous unfractionated heparin and stop 4 hours before surgery.
e. Give low-dose (prophylactic dose) subcutaneous low molecular weight heparin, administering the last dose 24 hours before surgery.

G2

A patient presents on your list for resection of an abdominal tumour of unknown aetiology.

Which of the following is most likely to be associated with a diagnosis of carcinoid disease?
a. Pulmonary fibrosis
b. Mixed mitral/aortic valve disease
c. Intermittent flushing
d. Recurrent constipation
e. Liver failure

G3

A 23-year-old woman with myasthenia gravis is scheduled for thymectomy. She was diagnosed 3 years ago and currently has an FVC of 3.5 l. She is seen regularly in clinic, and is compliant with medical advice.

Which of the following statements is most likely to be *true*?
a. The patient has a thymoma
b. A fibre-optic laryngoscope is likely to be required

Practice Single Best Answer Questions for the Final FRCA, ed. Hozefa Ebrahim, Khalid Hasan, Mark Tindall, Michael Clarke and Natish Bindal. Published by Cambridge University Press. © Cambridge University Press 2013.

c. A non-depolarizing muscle relaxant will be required to facilitate intubation
d. The patient will require prolonged postoperative ventilation
e. The patient will require premedication with an oral benzodiazepine

G4

Obstructive sleep apnoea is associated with the following physiological changes, except:
a. Intracranial hypertension
b. Gastro-oesophageal reflux
c. Systemic hypertension
d. Cor pulmonale
e. Increased growth hormone

G5

A 100-kg 34-year-old male presents with a 35% full thickness burn. He is admitted to critical care. Renal function begins to deteriorate, and 48 hours after admission his creatinine has risen from 100 to 350. Hourly urine output has averaged 25 ml hr^{-1} for the past 24 hours.

According to the RIFLE classification of renal dysfunction, this represents:
a. Risk of kidney injury
b. Acute kidney injury
c. Acute renal failure
d. Loss of renal function (chronic renal failure)
e. End-stage renal failure

G6

You are asked to anaesthetize a 5-year-old with cerebral palsy for repeat insertion of grommets. His mother tells you that he has recently suffered from another 'chest infection'. He saw his general practitioner 14 days ago with fever and a productive cough, and was treated with a course of antibiotics that finished 7 days ago. At present, he is apyrexial, his cough is much better, and non-productive. On examination, he has some quiet, bilateral wheeze, which clears with coughing.

What is the most appropriate course of action?
a. Discuss increased risks with parents and proceed to anaesthesia if they give consent
b. Postpone the case for 4–6 weeks
c. Use an ETT instead of an LMA to protect the airway from excess secretions
d. Use anticholinergics to reduce airway secretions
e. Use a bronchodilator nebulizer prior to anaesthesia

G7

A 22-year-old active cross-country runner presents for an open reduction and internal fixation of a non-united ankle fracture. Despite immobilization for 8 weeks and administration of paracetamol, ibuprofen and codeine in appropriate doses, the patient complains of severe pain in the foot. The foot is cool with smooth skin and obvious allodynia and hyperalgesia.

The most likely diagnosis is:
a. Complex regional pain syndrome (CRPS) type-2
b. Deep peroneal neuropathy

c. Ankle osteitis
d. Anterior tibial neuropathy
e. Complex regional pain syndrome (CRPS) type-1

G8

You are called urgently to an in-hospital cardiac arrest. On arrival, the team leader tells you the patient is asystolic in the third cycle of CPR. A 1-mg Minijet of adrenaline was administered down the ET tube a couple of minutes ago due to the lack of iv access. You manage to site a cannula.

What is the most appropriate next step?
a. Administer adrenaline 1 mg iv and atropine 3 mg iv before the fourth cycle of CPR
b. Administer adrenaline 1 mg and continue CPR
c. Pause to reassess the rhythm, and administer a DC shock if appropriate
d. Administer adrenaline 1 mg iv and atropine 3 mg iv and continue CPR.
e. Administer adrenaline 1 mg iv before the fourth cycle of CPR

G9

You are asked to review a 4-year-old child who is brought to A&E by his mother. She found him with an open box of aspirin tablets on the bathroom floor. She immediately brought the child to hospital, but it is now approximately 2 hours since the event. The child has vomited once and is pyrexial. His mother believes there are 28 missing tablets.

Which of the following investigations would best allow you to immediately assess the severity of the overdose?
a. Plasma salicylate levels
b. Blood gas analysis
c. Urine testing
d. Blood glucose level
e. ECG

G10

Which of the following statements regarding neuropathic pain is true?
a. Sensitization of nociceptors is a known mechanism of neuropathic pain
b. Chronic neuropathic pain should be suspected in a patient without neurological dysfunction
c. Persistent low mood can lead to neuropathic pain
d. Neuropathic pain can be a result of decreased activity of the serotonin receptors
e. Dynamic allodynia, sensory loss and hyperalgesia in an injury which is 3 weeks old classifies as chronic neuropathic pain

G11

You are called to urgently review a 35-year-old lady who is intubated and ventilated on the ICU. She was admitted following a high-speed road traffic collision in which she sustained head, chest and lower limb injuries. She has acutely desaturated to 80% on F_iO_2 100% and has become cardiovascularly unstable. Whilst reviewing her notes, you notice that she has not been prescribed low molecular weight heparin and consider a diagnosis of acute pulmonary embolism.

Which of the following would be the next most suitable investigation to confirm this?
a. Portable AP chest X-ray
b. 12-lead ECG
c. CTPA
d. D-dimer
e. Transthoracic echocardiogram

G12

A 45-year-old man has been removed from a furniture warehouse fire with signs of smoke inhalation and superficial burns to his legs. On arrival in the emergency department, he is breathless and drowsy. Initial arterial blood gas analysis demonstrates a profound metabolic acidosis with measured carbon monoxide levels of 12%.

Which of the following diagnoses and initial treatments is most appropriate?
a. Acute alcohol intoxication – gastric lavage
b. Carbon monoxide poisoning – hyperbaric therapy
c. Hypovolaemic shock – fluid resuscitation
d. Cyanide poisoning – 100% oxygen
e. Intracerebral event – rapid CT

G13

A 20-year-old male patient intubated and ventilated on ICU following a head injury requires brainstem death testing for potential organ donation.

Which of the following statements is *true*?
a. The pupils must be fixed and dilated
b. Lack of limb movement is essential
c. Two consultants must perform the tests
d. Caloric tests must be performed bilaterally
E. There must be no EEG activity

G14

You are asked to anaesthetize a 48-year-old lady, with a history of cirrhosis of the liver secondary to chronic hepatitis B infection, for an incarcerated umbilical hernia. She has signs of portal hypertension with ascites and splenomegaly. She has a haemoglobin of 8.6 g/dl, an INR of 1.6, with platelets of 80. Her sodium is 129 mmol/l, urea is 10.3 and creatinine is 129. Her LFTs reveal a bilirubin of 54 µmol/l, AST of 122 U/l, ALT of 98 U/l, alkaline phosphatase of 120 U/l and an albumin of 26 g/l.

What is your main priority for her anaesthetic management plan?
a. Correction of the coagulopathy and employment of a regional anaesthetic technique, to avoid the risk of volatile anaesthetics upon hepatic function
b. A rapid sequence induction to secure her airway followed by a general anaesthetic technique that maximizes hepatic oxygen delivery and perfusion, whilst minimizing hepatotoxicity
c. Cross-matching her for blood and fresh frozen plasma in case she bleeds

d. Delaying the case until she has been reviewed and optimized by the physicians
e. Judicious fluid management with sodium restriction, but taking care to preserve intravascular volume and urine output

G15

A 25-year-old female presents to the pain clinic following a normal laparoscopy. Her complaints include pelvic pain, menstrual pain and dyspareunia for 6 months. Examination is unremarkable. She is taking simple analgesics, but these are not effective.

Which diagnosis is least likely to explain her symptoms?
a. Vulvodynia
b. Irritable bowel syndrome
c. Endometriosis
d. Pelvic floor myalgia
e. Uterine retroversion

G16

You are performing a preoperative anaesthetic assessment for a patient with cirrhotic liver disease due to undergo an abdominal hysterectomy
Which of the following is most accurate?
a. A search for gallstones is indicated in case the cirrhosis is due to extrahepatic bile duct obstruction
b. A coagulation screen is the most sensitive indicator for the degree of hepatocellular dysfunction
c. The model for end-stage liver disease (MELD) score is indicated to predict perioperative risk
d. Serum blood must be checked for blood urea nitrogen
e. Hypoalbuminaemia should be corrected prior to surgery

G17

A consultant colleague has confessed to an addiction to alcohol. She has been informed by the General Medical Council that her work must be 'closely supervised by a registered medical practitioner of consultant grade'.

What is the meaning of 'closely supervised'?
a. She must be supervised as if she is a Foundation Year 1 doctor
b. She must be supervised as if she is a novice anaesthetist
c. She must be supervised as if she has 2–3 years anaesthetic experience
d. She must be supervised as if she is a final-year registrar
e. She doesn't need in-theatre supervision, but she must have regular meetings with another consultant to discuss her cases.

G18

Massive antepartum haemorrhage is a major cause of mortality and occurs with a frequency around 7 per 1000 deliveries. This equates to around 35 cases per year in a unit with 5000 deliveries per year. Antepartum haemorrhage is dangerous to both mother and foetus. Prompt recognition and treatment is essential. Team working between the specialties – obstetricians, haematologists and anaesthetists among others, is important and a knowledge of the various causes and outcomes of antepartum haemorrhage is vital to effective treatments.

a. Vasa praevia represents a serious threat to the mother if normal vaginal delivery is allowed to proceed.
b. Antepartum haemorrhage is only rarely a threat to the fetus
c. Over-estimation of blood loss leads to frequent unnecessary blood transfusions
d. In placenta praevia the first episode of bleeding is usually the most severe
e. Bleeding due to placental abruption is generally associated with more pain than bleeding due to placenta praevia

G19

The NAP3 study took place to determine the incidence of complications of central neuraxial block (CNB).

What was the quoted pessimistic risk of permanent harm or death in the chronic pain population following epidural CNB (cases per 100 000)?
a. 0
b. 0.6
c. 1.5
d. 2.6
e. 17.4

G20

A term baby delivered by Caesarean section is pale, blue and floppy. The midwife dries and stimulates the baby. Then she opens the airway but the baby does not breathe. She auscultates the heart rate and it is 50 bpm.

What should she do next?
a. Call the paediatrician to intubate the trachea
b. Site an iv cannula
c. Administer atropine at 20 mcg/kg
d. Commence chest compressions
e. Give five inflation breaths with a self-inflating bag and mask

G21

A 56-year-old man presents for an oesophagectomy for a squamous cell carcinoma. The surgeon decides to do this using a minimally invasive technique. During the laparoscopic part of the procedure, the airway pressure rises from 38 cmH$_2$O to 52 cmH$_2$O. There is evidence of decreased air entry on the left side.

The most likely cause of this is:
a. Intubation of the right main bronchus.
b. Capnothorax due to rapid passage of CO$_2$ into the left side of the chest from the abdomen through the surgical site.
c. Pulmonary metastases leading to lobar collapse
d. Pneumothorax secondary to high airway pressures
e. Pulmonary embolism in a patient who, due to the presence of malignancy, is in a prothrombotic state.

G22

You are the on-call obstetric anaesthetist and you are called to triage to see a primiparous woman at 34 weeks with pre-eclampsia. She needs a category 1 Caesarean section for foetal distress. Her most recent blood tests, taken last week, are as follows: Hb 12, WCC 5.6, platelets 80, her blood pressure is 150/92, she is taking labetalol and she last ate about half an hour ago.

What would your initial anaesthetic management plan be?
a. Spinal anaesthesia
b. Combined spinal–epidural anaesthesia
c. General anaesthesia with rapid sequence induction using alfentanil 1–2 mg, thiopentone 5 mg/kg and suxamethonium 1.5 mg/kg
d. Magnesium sulphate 4 g intravenously
e. Oral ranitidine and 15 l/min of oxygen via a facemask

G23

Which of the following is a clinical prediction scoring tool to assess the probability of deep vein thrombosis (DVT)?
a. TIMI risk score
b. Wells score
c. Wilson's score
d. euroSCORE
e. Framingham risk score

G24

Although ultrasound is becoming more commonly available, nerve stimulators are still used in a wide variety of peripheral nerve blocks. Correct use of the nerve stimulator increases the likelihood of a successful block and reduces the likelihood of injury to the patient.

Which of the following is true?
a. Muscle twitches associated with a current of over 3 mA imply intraneural needle placement
b. Electrode positioning is unimportant as long as a circuit is maintained
c. Large motor fibres have shorter chronaxy
d. If specific equipment is not available, the 'train of four' stimulator can be used instead
e. A pulse frequency of 20 Hz or greater is useful in locating motor nerves

G25

You have been asked to review a patient on the cardiac intensive care unit who is bleeding following a coronary artery bypass graft procedure. A thromboelastogram (TEG) to assess the patient's clotting shows: R-time 13 s (10–14 s); K-time 4 s (3–6 s); α-angle 50° (54–67°); MA 47 mm (59–68 mm). Lysis 30 is normal. The TEG is repeated with heparinase, and the results are the same.

Which of the following products would be most suitable to give in this case?
a. Platelets
b. Protamine
c. Tranexamic acid

d. Cryoprecipitate
e. Fresh frozen plasma

G26

Herbal remedies are often taken by patients alongside prescribed medication. Increased risk of bleeding is one of the effects of some herbal remedies.

Which of the following herbal remedies is not known to increase the risk of bleeding?
a. Echinacea
b. Garlic
c. Ginseng
d. Gingko biloba
e. Ginger

G27

A 34-year-old male presents for a shoulder arthroscopy. He is known to have bipolar disorder and is on lithium. He is otherwise fit and well.

Your anaesthetic plan would include most importantly:
a. The recommendation to stop lithium 24 hours preoperatively
b. Reduced doses of induction agents and reduced minimum alveolar concentration (MAC)
c. The use of neuromuscular monitoring or the avoidance of neuromuscular blocking drugs
d. Avoidance of NSAIDs
e. 5-lead ECG monitoring

G28

Intra-aortic balloon pump (IABP) increases the oxygen delivery to the myocardium and decreases the myocardial oxygen demand, thereby improving its function, especially in heart failure.

Which of the following physiological effects are not seen with a well-functioning IABP?
a. ↑ Aortic diastolic pressure
b. ↓ Left ventricle end-diastolic pressure
c. ↑ Coronary blood flow
d. ↓ Renal blood flow
e. ↓ Haemoglobin levels by up to 5%

G29

You are asked to anaesthetize a 60-year-old lady suffering from severe refractory depression for electro-convulsive therapy.

Which of the following induction agents would enable the greatest seizure quality?
a. Propofol
b. Etomidate
c. Thiopentone
d. Sevoflurane
e. Ketamine

G30

There are many hazards of providing anaesthesia for magnetic resonance imaging (MRI).

Which is of greatest concern to the anaesthetist?
a. Limited patient access and visibility
b. Interference or malfunctioning of monitoring equipment
c. Eddy currents in ECG leads may cause burns to the patient
d. Ferromagnetic objects may become projectile
e. Noise levels may make it difficult to hear monitoring alarms

Chapter 7

Paper G – Answers

G1

Answer: b.

The American College of Chest Physicians (ACCP) published revised guidelines on the management of perioperative anticoagulation and antiplatelet therapy in 2008. These guidelines attempt to strike a balance between the risk of thromboembolism and the risk of haemorrhage.

These guidelines divide each of the main indications for anticoagulation (mechanical heart valves, atrial fibrillation and thromboembolic disease) into three risk categories (high, medium and low risk) according to the probability of thromboembolism. Any mitral valve prosthesis, for example, is considered high-risk. The guidelines recommend that high-risk patients should receive 'bridging' anticoagulation whilst not covered by vitamin K antagonists. First choice is high-dose low molecular weight heparin (LMWH) continuing up to 24 hours before surgery. Unfractionated heparin by infusion up to 4 hours before surgery is considered an acceptable alternative, but much less convenient. Low-dose LMWH would not be considered sufficient for high-risk patients.

Oral anticoagulants may be safely restarted 12–24 hours after surgery since the time to peak effect is delayed. High-dose LMWH may be delayed until 48–72 hours post procedure to mitigate bleeding concerns.

Discontinuing anticoagulants without implementing bridging therapy would be inappropriate for this patient, since he is at high risk of thromboembolic phenomena. A 4-hour delay between high-dose LMWH and surgery is too short due to the haemorrhagic risk involved.

Douketis JD, Berger PB, Dunn AS, *et al.* The perioperative management of antithrombotic therapy: American College of Chest Physicians evidence-based clinical practice guidelines (8th edn). *Chest* 2008; **133**: 299S–339S

G2

Answer: c.

Tumours of enterochromaffin cells give rise to carcinoid disease. Primaries are most commonly located in the small bowel, but may also originate from the stomach, appendix or distal colon/rectum. Less commonly, they arise from the bronchopulmonary tree.

Practice Single Best Answer Questions for the Final FRCA, ed. Hozefa Ebrahim, Khalid Hasan, Mark Tindall, Michael Clarke and Natish Bindal. Published by Cambridge University Press. © Cambridge University Press 2013.

Carcinoid disease encompasses many different neuroendocrine cell tumours, which typically secrete several possible biogenic amines. Classically, this predominantly involves 5-hydroxytryptophan, but can also include other vasoactive mediators, such as histamine, dopamine and kallikrein. These can be released in response to exercise, and by certain foods such as alcohol and tyramine-containing foods (cheese). If they escape into the general circulation, they can result in flushing episodes (particularly of the upper body) or 'carcinoid syndrome', as well as other symptoms such as diarrhoea or bronchospasm. These mediators are metabolized by the liver and so the carcinoid syndrome is only seen if the tumour is located outside the portal venous drainage system or if it has metastasized to the liver or distantly. Unless there is massive liver involvement, hepatic failure is rare. Chronically high systemic serotonin (5-HT) levels result in characteristic right-sided heart disease, which can be severe. There is endocardial fibrosis, fibrosis and tethering of the tricuspid and pulmonary valves and right-sided diastolic dysfunction. Left-sided heart failure is atypical. Pulmonary fibrosis is not normally seen. Bronchospasm as a result of carcinoid syndrome may occur, or direct obstructive bronchogenic lesions can cause pneumonias or lung collapse.

Powell B, Al Mukhtar, A, Mills GH. Carcinoid: the disease and its implications for anaesthesia. *Contin Educ Anaesth Crit Care* 2011; **11**(1): 9–13

G3

Answer: c.

About 15% of patients with myasthenia gravis (MG) have thymomas. Thymectomy is now recommended in all adults with MG; the presence of a thymoma is not a requirement for surgery.

The most common approach is transsternal. Few patients actually require prolonged postoperative ventilation even after sternotomy.

While profound weakness would allow intubation without relaxation, perioperative management with anticholinesterases often means that most patients do require some degree of neuromuscular block to allow endotracheal intubation. Non-depolarizing muscle relaxants are not contra-indicated; however, their effects may be profound and therefore monitoring of blockade should be considered mandatory.

Bogaert F, Verhaeghen D, Herregods L. Myasthenia gravis and thymectomy: an anaesthetic approach. *Acta Anaesth Belg* 2007; **58**: 185–190
Thavasothy M, Hirsch N. Myasthenia gravis. *Contin Educ Anaesth Crit Care* 2002; **2**(3): 88–90

G4

Answer: e.

Obstructive sleep apnoea (OSA) affects an increasing number of people in the UK. The prevalence is 5%–10% in the adult population, but it can also affect children. It is a multisystem disorder, but the primary drive is the presence of a reversible blockade to air flow of the naso/oropharynx during sleep. Excessive bony and/or soft tissue overgrowth accentuates the normal physiological relaxation of the pharyngeal muscles during sleep and causes hypoventilation or apnoea. This is normally followed by arousal (caused by decreasing pO_2 ± increasing pCO_2) and resolution of the obstruction. This occurs repeatedly during sleep. Frequent arousals and disruption of sleep lead to daytime somnolence, but also to anxiety and depression, and patients can develop chronic headache and intracranial hypertension. Over time, repeated episodes of hypoxaemia, and the hypertension associated with arousal episodes, cause other physiological changes. Systemic hypertension develops either as a consequence of the disease or the poor health causing the disease. Pulmonary hypertension is common and can eventually result in cor pulmonale as the right heart cannot cope with the increased afterload. The endocrine system may also be involved. Diabetes is more common and often blood sugar control is difficult. There can also be a reduction in growth hormone and testosterone levels leading to growth retardation in children. There is an increased risk of gastro-oesophageal reflux disease.

Martinez G, Faber P. Obstructive sleep apnoea. *Contin Educ Anaesth Crit Care Pain* 2011; **11**(1): 5–8

G5

Answer: c.

Classification	Degree of functional loss	Reduction in urine output
Risk	25% decrease in GFR or 1.5 × increase in creatinine	< 0.5 ml/kg/hr for 6 hours
Injury	50% decrease in GFR or 2.0 × increase in creatinine	< 0.5 ml/kg/hr for 12 hours
Failure	75% decrease in GFR or 3.0 × increase in creatinine	< 0.3 ml/kg/hr for 24 hours / anuria for 12 hours
Loss	Complete loss of renal function for > 4 weeks	
End stage	Complete loss of renal function for > 3 months	

Webb S, Allen J. Perioperative renal protection. *Contin Educ Anaesth Crit Care Pain* 2008; **8**: 176–180

G6

Answer: a.

This is a commonly encountered, difficult situation. The concern with recent upper respiratory tract infection (URTI) is an increased risk of respiratory complications, particularly laryngospasm, bronchospasm and hypoxia. These risks are approximately ten-fold compared with the healthy child, extend for up to 6 weeks after resolution of symptoms and are particularly associated with the use of an endotracheal tube (ETT) rather than a laryngeal mask airway (LMA). Traditionally, all children should be postponed for 4–6 weeks following an URTI to allow complete resolution of symptoms.

It is easy to decide to anaesthetize a child with a URTI who requires urgent surgery, or to anaesthetize a child who is fully recovered from a URTI. Equally, it is easy to cancel a poorly child with a fever, or purulent sputum, who requires non-urgent surgery.

Most cases fall somewhere in-between; usually a child needs minor day-case surgery (dental extraction, tonsillectomy, circumcision), has had a cold recently, but is back to 'his normal self', with no fever, but some residual nasal congestion or dry cough. In fact, many children can go through a whole winter without ever being entirely free of URTI symptoms, especially children with underlying respiratory or neurological diseases.

A pragmatic approach is therefore required. The risk of respiratory complications is higher. However, these risks will still be low overall. Scandanavian studies from the 1980s showed a five-fold increase in the risk of laryngospasm (96/1000 cf. 17/1000) and a ten-fold increase in the risk of bronchospasm (41/1000 cf. 4/1000). It is likely that these risks have fallen further as knowledge and techniques evolve.

Avoiding an ETT is possible (many dental extractions can be performed with an LMA *in situ*). Anticholinergics may reduce secretions and bronchodilators may reduce wheeze, but if these drugs are required, this may indicate significant ongoing pathology, and postponement may be prudent.

A risk–benefit analysis should be performed for each case, and the risks discussed with the parent(s). Fever, purulent sputum, leukocytosis and X-ray changes would usually be considered contra-indications to general anaesthesia for elective surgery. However, a blanket policy cancelling all patients with URTI symptoms for fear of fatal respiratory complications is unfounded. Most children recovering from URTI, or with mild symptoms would be expected to undergo general anaesthesia without any significant problems.

Cote CJ. Preoperative preparation and premedication. *Br J Anaesth* 1999; **83**: 16–28
Tait AR, Malviya S. Anesthesia for the child with an upper respiratory tract infection: still a dilemma? *Anesth Analge* 2005; **100**(1): 59–65

G7

Answer: e.

CRPS type-2 is associated with an obvious nerve injury. Pain is not in a clear nerve distribution of either the anterior tibial or deep peroneal nerves, despite these nerves lying in close proximity to the ankle joint. This case is typical of CRPS type 1 with a pain duration exceeding the expected duration from the injury, temperature difference, early evidence of atrophy and sensory nerve dysfunction.

- *Allodynia*: painful sensation from a non-painful stimulus
- *Hyperalgesia*: exaggerated response to a painful stimulus

Shipton EA. Complex regional pain syndrome – Mechanisms, diagnosis, and management. *Curr Anaesth Crit Care* 2009; **20**: 209–214.

G8

Answer: b.

The Resuscitation Council UK Algorithm (2010) for non-shockable rhythms should be followed for asystolic and PEA cardiac arrests.

Compared with the 2005 guidelines, the endotracheal route is no longer recommended for drug delivery, and atropine is no longer recommended for routine use in PEA/asystole. 1 mg iv adrenaline should be given as soon as cardiac arrest is confirmed. However, the timing of subsequent doses for shockable rhythms has changed. In 2005, 1 mg was given just before the third shock, now it is recommended to be given after the third shock, just after chest compressions have resumed. This is to allow more prompt defibrillation and minimize the interruptions to chest compressions.

In general, the changes in the 2010 guidelines aim to emphasize high-quality, uninter-rupted chest compressions, and de-emphasize the importance of intubation of the trachea.

Resuscitation Council (UK). *Adult Advanced Life Support: Online.* Available at: http://www.resus.org.uk/pages/als.pdf. Accessed 14/02/2012

G9

Answer: b.

Aspirin is a common drug involved in cases of accidental poisoning in children. Ingestions of <150 mg/kg are considered non-toxic; patients who take 150–300 mg/kg exhibit signs of mild to moderate toxicity and can be treated by rehydration. Ingestions of >500 mg/kg, as described in this case, are considered potentially life threatening.

Children do not usually display the respiratory alkalosis associated with adult salicylate overdose. Symptoms of acute toxicity develop more rapidly and are more severe in children than adults. Children often present with nausea and vomiting followed by tinnitus or deafness and fever. Fits, coma, hypotension and pulmonary oedema may be seen as acid-aemia progresses and severe fluid and electrolyte imbalances occur. Hypoglycaemia is common in this setting and must be guarded against. For this reason, point-of-care analysis of acid–base balance and serum electrolytes would be the next most appropriate investiga-tion; however, formal blood samples should also be sent to the laboratory for assessment of serum electrolytes, renal and hepatic function, and blood glucose to confirm results.

Plasma drug levels (if available) should always be measured when exposure to toxins is suspected. Plasma salicylate concentrations should be measured at least 4 h after ingestion, therefore drug levels may not impact on management in acute poisoning. Similarly, bedside urine tests are of limited use: they are non-specific and do not give reliable results regarding the timing of exposure to the toxin. An ECG should be performed, which may detect conduction abnormalities of diagnostic and prognostic importance, however this would be a lower priority in this scenario.

Penny L, Moriarty T. Poisoning in children. *Contin Educ Anaesth Crit Care Pain* 2009; 9(4): 100–113

G10

Answer: a.

Neuropathic pain is defined as 'pain initiated or caused by a primary lesion or dysfunction of the nervous system' and a patient who does not have neurological dysfunction is unlikely to have neuropathic pain. Pain after surgery, diabetic neuropathy and pain due to multiple sclerosis are all known causes of neuropathic pain. Low mood usually occurs in patients suffering from neuropathic pain, but it does not cause it. Various mechanisms of neuro-pathic pain have been accepted, which are sensitization of nociceptors, NMDA receptor upregulation and increased sodium channel activation. Dynamic allodynia, sensory loss and hyperalgesia are all features of neuropathic pain but a pain history of less than 3 months is not described as chronic pain.

Merksey H, Bogduk N. *Classification of Chronic Pain: Descriptions of Chronic Pain Syndromes and Definitions of Pain Terms*, 2nd edn, 1994. Seattle: IASP Press.

Callin S, Bennett M. Assessment of neuropathic pain. *Contin Educ Anaesth Crit Care Pain* 2008; 8(6): 210–213

G11

Answer: e.

Classification of pulmonary thromboembolism (PTE) can be based on physiological grounds; a differentiation between massive, submassive, and non-massive pulmonary embolism has been proposed. Massive pulmonary embolism (5%) can cause haemodynamic instability (as in this case) and precipitate cardiopulmonary arrest. Emboli in this situation tend to be larger and there is demonstrable right ventricular dysfunction. Submassive pulmonary embolism (25%) is more difficult to demonstrate as patients tend to be haemodynamically stable.

Echocardiography is useful in assessing cardiac function at the bedside. In massive PTE, thrombus can occasionally be seen proximally in the main pulmonary artery. More commonly, it is the effect on the right side of the heart that can be seen, i.e. dilated right atrium/right ventricle and impaired right ventricular function. Routine use of echo is, however, not advised for all suspected cases of PTE at present, and should be reserved for unstable patients with suspected massive and submassive PTE who cannot be safely transported to the radiology department. Computerized tomographic pulmonary angiography (CTPA) is the radiological investigation of choice in stable patients with suspected non-massive PTE.

ECG, chest X-ray (CXR) and D-dimer have insufficient sensitivity or specificity, even when used in association with clinical assessment to exclude a diagnosis of PTE. The classical S1Q3T3 pattern on ECG is a non-specific sign of acute right heart strain and occurs in <20% of patients with PTE. CXR in pulmonary embolism can demonstrate hypovascularity or an area of pleural-based wedge-shaped consolidation suggesting infarction. In hospitalized patients, D-dimer has little value, as most will have underlying diseases or postoperative states that cause increased plasma levels.

van Beek, JR, Elliot CA, Kiely DG. Diagnosis and initial treatment of patients with suspected pulmonary thromboembolism. *Contin Educ Anaesth Crit Care Pain* 2009; **9** (4): 119–124

G12

Answer: d.

Cyanide is released from burning polyurethane foam. Upon inhalation, it inhibits cellular cytochrome oxidase, blocking the tricarboxylic acid cycle and stopping cellular respiration. Acute poisoning causes dizziness, headache, palpitations, breathlessness, drowsiness, coma, convulsions, pulmonary oedema and metabolic acidosis, all due to increasing hypoxia. These features would not be present at relatively low levels of carbon monoxide (<15%). The Health and Safety Executive no longer recommend a cyanide antidote, instead concentrating on supportive therapy including maximizing oxygen delivery.

> HSE will no longer recommend the use of any antidote in the first-aid treatment of cyanide poisoning and will not require employers to keep supplies. There is a great deal of anecdotal evidence of the value of oxygen and the experience of most occupational physicians is that the majority of victims of mild to moderate cyanide poisoning improve rapidly when treated with

oxygen alone. HSE will in future advise that administration of oxygen is the most useful initial treatment for cyanide poisoning

Health and Safety Executive. Cyanide poisoning – New recommendations on first aid treatment.

G13
Answer: d.

The UK code for the diagnosis of brainstem death has three essential components:

1. Fulfilment of essential preconditions
2. Exclusion of potentially reversible contributions to an apnoeic state
3. The formal demonstration of coma, apnoea, and the absence of brainstem reflex activity

The tests should be carried out by two doctors competent with the procedure. One must be a consultant and the other registered with the GMC for at least 5 years. The tests must be performed by the doctors together and two sets of tests must be completed.

The preconditions are:

1. Apnoeic coma requiring ventilation
2. Irreversible brain damage of known aetiology, e.g. subarachnoid haemorrhage, ischaemic stroke, trauma

It must be ensured that the apnoeic coma is not due to reversible influences, such as hypothermia, metabolic disturbance, endocrine disturbance, sedative drugs or cardiovascular instability.

Once the preconditions have been met, formal testing can take place. Family members should be given the opportunity to witness the tests. The brainstem tests and cranial nerves tested are shown below:

Test	Cranial nerve	
	Sensory	Motor
Pupillary response	II	III
Corneal reflexes	V	VII
Oculovestibular reflexes	VIII	III, IV, VI
Response to painful stimulus	V	VII
Gag reflex	IX	X
Cough reflex	X	X

Pupil size is not important, but direct and consensual reflexes should be absent. Spinal reflexes may be present so limb movement can occur in a brainstem dead patient, but not within the cranial distribution. Caloric testing should occur bilaterally, but inability to perform the test on one side does not invalidate the test. The apnoea test should only be performed once the total absence of brainstem activity has been demonstrated.

An EEG can be used as an ancillary test under certain circumstances, such as when a comprehensive neurological examination cannot be performed, for example due to facial trauma, but it is not required to make the diagnosis of brainstem death.

For children over 2 months of age, brainstem death is diagnosed in the same way as adults. Below this age, the preconditions for testing are rarely met.

Oram J, Murphy P. Diagnosis of death. *Contin Educ Anaesth Crit Care Pain* 2011; **11**(3): 77–81

Academy of the Medical Royal Colleges. *A Code of Practice for the Diagnosis and Confirmation of Death*. London, 2008.

G14

Answer: b.

While e. is also a true answer, and arguably c., they are not the *main* priorities for her anaesthetic management.

Steadman R. Anaesthesia for liver transplant surgery. *Anesthesiology Clin N Am* 2004; **22**(4): 687–711

Morgan GE, Mikhail MS. *Clinical Anesthesiolgy*, 4th edn, 2006. USA: McGraw-Hill, 797–801

G15

Answer: e.

Chronic pelvic pain (CPP) is non-malignant pain perceived in structures related to the pelvis in men and women. There is often a poor correlation between identifiable pathology and severity of pain. A laparoscopy is often carried out to exclude infection, malignancy or any obvious pathology. Laparoscopies frequently do not reveal any abnormality or a reason for the pain. A normal laparoscopy does not exclude endometriosis or pelvic floor myalgia and a normal examination does not exclude vulvodynia. Uterine retroversion is very common and can cause mechanical pelvic pain. It is usually diagnosed by clinical examination and seen on laparoscopy. All the disorders listed could present with pelvic pain, menstrual pain and dyspareunia, though not all have a gynaecological aetiology. Pathology of the urinary tract, gastrointestinal tract, neurological and musculoskeletal system can all present in this way. CPP is a complex pain problem, which can severely disrupt quality of life. Once assessed and investigated, CPP is best managed in an interdisciplinary fashion if a surgical explanation is not found.

Fall M, Baranowski AP, Elneil S *et al*. EUA guidelines on chronic pelvic pain. *Europ Urol* 2010; **57**(1): 35–48

G16

Answer: b.

Although the MELD score has been demonstrated to predict survival in patients undergoing transjugular intrahepatic porto-systemic shunting, large prospective studies in cirrhotic patients undergoing non-hepatic surgeries are lacking. Blood urea nitrogen may be useful in some patients, but is not indicated routinely.

Steadman R. Anaesthesia for liver transplant surgery. *Anesthesiology Clin N Am* 2004; **22**(4): 687–711

Morgan GE, Mikhail MS. *Clinical Anesthesiolgy*, 4th edn, 2006. USA: McGraw-Hill, 797–801

G17

Answer: b.

The GMC can place restrictions on a doctor's registration following problems with addiction. The terminology can read 'directly supervised', which requires supervision equivalent to an FY1, 'closely supervised', which requires supervision equivalent to a novice anaesthetist or 'supervised', which means supervision equivalent to that of a middle grade trainee.

AAGBI *Drug and Alcohol Abuse Amongst Anaesthetists 2 – Guidance on Identification and Management*, 2011

G18

Answer: e.

Vasa praevia refers to a velamentous insertion of the umbilical cord where the fetal vessels traverse the fetal membranes ahead of the presenting part. Rupture of these vessels carries very little risk to the mother but a grave risk of fetal exsanguination.

Most forms of antepartum haemorrhage present a greater risk to the fetus than to the mother due to the smaller circulating volume of the latter and the lack of obvious symptoms of fetal blood loss.

Under-estimation of blood loss is a danger in all situations. Even measurement of haemoglobin does not guarantee accurate assessment because whole blood is lost and so haemoglobin does not change acutely. Assessment of blood loss requires many factors to be borne in mind and, if ongoing blood loss is likely, it may be wise to have a high index of suspicion and, if haemoglobin is to be the trigger, then it may be wise to transfuse at a higher haemoglobin than usual. Be aware that a situation that seems to be under control can very rapidly tumble out of control with potentially catastrophic consequences. Seek help early – particularly if help is far away.

Banks A, Norris A. Massive haemorrhage in pregnancy. *Contin Educ Anaesth Crit Care Pain* 2005; 5(6): 195–198

Gupta R, Kilby M, Cooper G. Fetal surgery and anaesthetic implications. *Contin Educ Anaesth Crit Care Pain* 2008; 8(2): 71–75

Thomas C, Madej T. Obstetric emergencies and the anaesthetist. *Contin Educ Anaesth Crit Care Pain* 2002; 2(6): 174–177

G19

Answer: a.

The NAP3 study was designed to answer the following questions:

- What types of CNB are used in the UK and how often?
- How often do major complications, leading to permanent harm, occur in association with CNB?
- What happens to the patients experiencing these complications?

Due to clinical uncertainty regarding some of the reported cases, particularly in regard to final outcome, the results were quoted as a pessimistic and optimistic incidence. During the

12 months studied, there were over 700 000 CNBs performed. The incidence of permanent injury due to CNB (expressed per 100 000 cases) was pessimistically 4.2 and optimistically 2.0. These are equivalent to 1 in 24 000 and 1 in 54 000 respectively and are considerably lower than had been previously suggested.

In the 30 patients with permanent harm, 60% occurred after epidural block, 23% after spinal block and 13% after a combined spinal–epidural (CSE) block. More than 80% of these patients had a CNB placed for perioperative analgesia.

Perioperative epidurals represented 1 in 7 of all CNB, but accounted for more than half of complications leading to harm. CSEs represented less than 6% of all CNBs, but accounted for more than 13% of cases leading to harm.

Of particular note was the failure to identify and understand the relevance of inappropriately weak legs after CNB.

There were no cases of permanent harm reported following an epidural for chronic pain, though of course this does not equate to the absence of risk. The report highlighted that chronic pain patients are usually discharged the same day and that they should be discharged with written advice concerning what to do should a complication arise.

Cook TM, Counsell D, Wildsmith JA. Major complications of central neuraxial block: report on the Third National Audit Project of the Royal College of Anaesthetists. *Br J Anaesth* 2009; **102**(2): 179–190

G20

Answer: e.

Bradycardia in this situation is usually secondary to hypoxia. The baby has not taken its first breath yet and thus its lungs will be full of fluid. The inflation breaths should last 2–3 seconds each and reach a pressure of 30 cmH$_2$O. Inflation of the lungs and subsequent oxygenation should lead to a rapid rise in heart rate.

Atropine, whilst a treatment for bradycardia, will not resolve the underlying cause of hypoxia. Intubation is not required to attempt the five inflation breaths, which can be delivered via a facemask. Should the baby remain bradycardic following five successful inflation breaths, chest compressions may be commenced.

2010 Resuscitation Guidelines. *Newborn Life Support*. www.resus.org.uk

G21

Answer: d.

Intubation of the right main bronchus is a possibility, particularly if there has been a recent change in position; however, this is not mentioned in the question. Pulmonary embolism and pulmonary metastases would not cause acute and widespread reduction of air entry with rising airway pressures as seen in this setting. The minimally invasive oesophagectomy technique does involve creating a surgical communication between the abdomen and chest through which CO$_2$ from the laparoscopic element of the procedure can pass. However, this is not as common a clinical presentation as pneumothorax secondary to high airway pressures during the laparoscopy.

Rucklidge M, Sanders D, Martin A. Anaesthesia for minimally invasive oesophagectomy. *Contin Educ Anaesth Crit Care Pain* 2010; **10**(2), 43–47.

G22

Answer: c.

The Caesarean section rate for England and Wales is 21%. Despite this, the incidence of general anaesthesia for Caesarean section is decreasing because of the use of regional anaesthesia in the majority of cases.

The common indications for general anaesthesia for Caesarean section are urgency, maternal refusal of regional techniques, inadequate or failed regional techniques and regional contra-indications such as coagulation or spinal abnormalities. Obstetric indications such as placenta praevia are no longer considered absolute indications for general anaesthesia.

In this case the main contra-indication to regional anaesthesia is the low platelet count in the context of pre-eclampsia. A more recent platelet count should ideally be available, but as there is insufficient time in this scenario it would be prudent to avoid a regional technique.

The complications of general anaesthesia include failed intubation, aspiration, awareness and increased blood loss.

McGlennan A, Mustafa A. General anaesthesia for Caesarean section. *Contin Educ Anaesth Crit Care Pain* 2009; **9**(5): 148–151

G23

Answer: b.

Deep vein thrombosis is an important disease process because it has two important sequelae: pulmonary embolus and the post-thrombotic syndrome (a disorder of chronic venous incompetence resulting in chronic pain, oedema, ulceration and hyperpigmentation). Early recognition is important to reduce the risk of complications developing. The Wells diagnostic algorithm is designed for this purpose. A DVT is likely if two or more of the following points exist, and unlikely if one or less is present. Two points are subtracted if another diagnosis is considered more likely than DVT.

- Active cancer (treatment ongoing or within the last 6 months)
- Paralysis, paresis or recent plaster immobilization of the legs
- Recently bedridden for more than 3 days, or major surgery within the last 12 weeks
- Localized tenderness along the distribution of the deep venous system (such as the back of the calf)
- Entire leg is swollen
- Calf swelling by more than 3 cm compared with the asymptomatic leg (measured 10 cm below the tibial tuberosity).
- Pitting oedema (greater than on the asymptomatic leg).
- Collateral superficial veins (non-varicose).
- Previously documented DVT.

The Thrombosis in Myocardial Infarction score stratifies risk in acute coronary syndromes. The Wilson's score predicts difficult endotracheal intubation. The euroSCORE is the European System for Cardiac Operative Risk Evaluation. The Framingham risk score estimates the 10-year cardiovascular risk of an individual.

Barker RC, Marval P. Venous thromboembolism: risks and prevention. *Contin Educ Anaesth Crit Care Pain* 2011; **11**(1): 18–23

G24

Answer: c.

Current delivered to the nerve from an electrical nerve locator is measured in amperes. The rheobase of a given nerve is the minimum current required to cause propagation of an impulse along the nerve. Chronaxy is the minimum time of application of a current of twice the rheobase that will cause an impulse to be propagated. Larger nerves have shorter chronaxy, so it is possible to stimulate motor fibres without stimulating pain fibres, as the latter are narrower and have longer chronaxy. Current is generally limited to around 1 mA. Twitches below 0.2 mA may indicate intraneural placement of the stimulating needle.

A frequency of 1 or 2 hertz is usually used to allow the operator to see twitches clearly. Higher frequencies are painful and may cause tetanic contractions of muscles.

Polarity is important. If the electrode nearest the nerve is the cathode, lower currents can be used because the flow of current causes the membrane of the adjacent nerve to depolarize. If the circuit is reversed, the membrane tends to hyperpolarize near the needle and depolarize further away. This arrangement is less efficient and requires much higher currents.

Dalrymple P, Chelliah S. Electrical nerve locators. *Contin Educ Anaesth Crit Care Pain* 2006; 6(1): 32–36

G25

Answer: a.

Thromboelastography (TEG) is a quick and easy bedside analysis of clotting, which is performed on whole blood. It provides information not only on the speed and strength of clot formation, but also on the degree of fibrinolysis, neither of which can be assessed using APTT or PT. A suspended wire is introduced into a small cuvette/cup of whole blood, which rotates and oscillates. As the blood begins to clot, movements of the cup are transmitted via the wire and translated into graphical form. This correlates with the viscoelastic properties of the clot formed.

The R-time is taken from the start of the test to initial fibrin formation. This correlates with APTT and PT; therefore a prolonged R-time indicates a deficiency in clotting factors or platelets or anticoagulation. The maximum amplitude (MA) represents the strength of the clot and is dependent on platelet count and function. K-time is the time taken for the graph to widen to 20 mm and represents fibrinogen formation and platelet function. The α-angle represents rate of fibrin build-up and cross-linking. Finally, lysis-30 measures the percentage of amplitude reduction 30 minutes after MA. This is a reflection of clot stability, i.e. degree of fibrinolysis.

The TEG in this example has a raised R-time, reduced α-angle and MA. The patient also has a prolonged activated clotting time (ACT). This would indicate a deficiency in clotting factors or platelets with the possibility of an anticoagulant effect. The repeat TEG with heparinase is designed to determine whether any of the abnormalities are due to heparin. Heparinase breaks down any heparin present, eliminating its effect. If this were the case, you would expect the TEG to normalize. However, there is no change in this situation, implying that the abnormal TEG is due to a true deficiency in clotting factors or platelets, so the correct treatment would be to give FFP and platelets. Tranexamic acid is an antifibrinolytic drug;

lysis 30 is normal, so fibrinolysis is normal. Cryoprecipitate is not required as the TEG does not indicate a deficiency of fibrinogen.

Mallett SV, Cox DJA. Thromboelastography: a review article. *Br J Anaesth* 1992; **69**: 307–313

G26

Answer: a.

Echinacea is thought to improve the immune system through cytokine modulation and may reduce the severity and duration of upper respiratory tract infections.

Whilst answers b.–e. are not always taken for their property of increased bleeding, they can all cause it. Garlic contains cysteine which reduces thromboxane formation and alters arachidonic acid metabolism. It inhibits platelet aggregation. Ginseng interferes with platelet aggregation. Gingko biloba is a potent inhibitor of platelet activating factor. Ginger is a potent inhibitor of thromboxane synthetase and can therefore prolong bleeding time.

Wong A, Townley S. Herbal medicines and anaesthesia. *Cont in Educ Anaesth Crit Care* 2011; **11**(1): 14–17

G27

Answer: c.

Lithium does not need to be stopped for minor surgery. There is dispute whether or not it should be stopped 24–48 hours before major surgery as, due to its effects on the brainstem, blocking the release of dopamine and noradrenaline, it may decrease anaesthetic requirements. However, the psychiatric implications of stopping and restarting lithium can lead to more mood disturbance than if the patient were left untreated. Lithium is additive with depolarizing block and synergistic with non-depolarizing neuromuscular blockade, causing prolongation of both; so neuromuscular monitoring must always be used. Lithium is renally excreted and has a narrow therapeutic window, so caution is required when potentially nephrotoxic drugs are used. Lithium has been associated with conduction defects under GA.

Flood S, Bodenham A. Lithium: mimicry, mania, and muscle relaxants. *Contin Educ Anaesth Crit Care Pain* 2010; **10**(3): 77–80

G28

Answer: d.

IABP not only improves the function of the left ventricle, but has a favourable effect on the right ventricle. The pressure gradient between the aorta and the left ventricle increases when the IABP balloon inflates during diastole. This increases the coronary blood flow, hence improving the oxygen delivery to the myocardium. During systole, the balloon deflates, which decreases the afterload of the left ventricle. The coronary blood flow in patients suffering from severe coronary artery disease depends directly on the diastolic perfusion pressure. Since the IABP increases the diastolic pressure, the coronary blood flow increases in these patients. The increased cardiac output improves the renal blood flow which may increase up to 25%. The urine output occasionally decreases after initiating the IABP, which may be due to inappropriate placement of the balloon. Haemolysis may decrease the haemoglobin levels and the haematocrit by up to 5%.

Krishna M, Zacharowski K. Principles of intra-aortic balloon pump counterpulsation. *Contin Educ Anaesth Crit Care Pain* 2009; **9**(1): 24–28

G29

Answer: b.

Doses of induction agents are initially titrated to a patient's weight. This may be modified on subsequent treatments as necessary, depending on previous response to ECT and changing seizure thresholds. Methohexital, which had minimal anticonvulsant properties compared with other barbiturates, was the original gold standard, but due initially to lack of availability, other hypnotic drugs have become more widely used.

A recent systematic review concluded that all currently available induction agents are suitable for ECT and the small variations in emergence and recovery times should not govern drug choice (ketamine, however, was not included).

Etomidate results in the longest seizure duration, and it is the only iv induction agent that may reduce the seizure threshold. Combining opioids such as remifentanil (1 µg/kg over 30–60 s) or alfentanil (10–25 µg/kg) with agents other than etomidate can produce similar effects on seizure duration by an induction agent dose-sparing effect. Whichever drug is used, it is preferable to utilize the same one throughout a course of treatment to avoid interfering with the seizure threshold (which generally increases over a course of ECT).

Uppal V, Dourish J, Macfarlane A. Anaesthesia for electroconvulsive therapy. *Contin Educ Anaesth Crit Care Pain* 2010; **10** (6); 192–196

G30

Answer: a.

This question highlights a number of challenges for the anaesthetist:

- Uncooperative patients with no insight or capacity to understand any planned intervention often require a GA for MRI
- An environment remote to theatre with staff who may be unfamiliar with the practice of anaesthesia and sedation
- A patient who may have complex co-existing disease
- Anaesthesia in a powerful magnetic field with its associated risks for the patients and staff
- Limited access to the patient during the procedure

Further information may be found in the following RCoA and AAGBI documents.

Royal College of Anaesthetists. *Guidance on Provision of Anaesthetic Care in the Non-theatre Environment*. Revised 2011
Association of Anaesthetists of Great Britain and Ireland Guideline. *Safety in Magnetic Resonance Units 2010 – An Update*. 2010

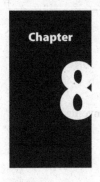

Chapter 8

Paper H – Questions

H1

You admit a patient to your intensive care unit, and require a venous thromboembolism (VTE) risk assessment as part of your normal hospital protocol.

Which of the following risk factors is not commonly linked to increased risk of VTE?
a. Congestive cardiac failure
b. Female sex
c. Lupus anticoagulant
d. Previous varicose vein surgery
e. Nephrotic syndrome

H2

The midwife looking after a 43-year-old, gravida-eight Afro-Caribbean lady notices she is bleeding PV postnatally.

Which of the following statements is most correct in assessing and managing this patient?
a. PPH is defined as the loss of 500 ml or more of blood from the genital tract within 24 hours of the birth of a baby
b. Risk factors for PPH include: previous PPH, Afro-Caribbean ethnicity, obesity (BMI>35) and anaemia
c. Allowing hypotension is acceptable to reduce the rate of blood loss
d. 4.5 litres of clear fluids is the maximum that should be infused whilst awaiting compatible blood
e. Administration of oxytocin infusion of 5 units diluted in 50 ml saline titrated up to 4 ml/h is indicated

H3

A 3-week-old baby boy with pyloric stenosis has undergone medical management and now presents for surgery.

Which of the following statements is true?
a. He must be induced using a rapid sequence induction
b. Pyloric stenosis is associated with significant congenital cardiac disease
c. He is likely to develop postoperative hypoglycaemia

Practice Single Best Answer Questions for the Final FRCA, ed. Hozefa Ebrahim, Khalid Hasan, Mark Tindall, Michael Clarke and Natish Bindal. Published by Cambridge University Press. © Cambridge University Press 2013.

165

d. He is unlikely to have postoperative apnoeas
e. He will have a persistent metabolic alkalosis

H4

A patient with lung cancer presents for pneumonectomy. The following investigations most accurately predict suitability for resection:
a. Preoperative FEV_1 >70% of predicted
b. Predicted post-operative FEV_1 <40% of preoperative
c. FEV_1 >1500 ml
d. FEV_1 >2000 ml
e. Maximal oxygen uptake (VO_2) of 12 ml/kg/min on cardiopulmonary exercise testing

H5

You are called to see a 65-year-old man in the emergency department. He presents with sudden onset of severe chest pain radiating to his back. His ECG shows ischaemic changes. His BP is 200/95 mmHg, HR 110/min. His chest X-ray shows a widened mediastinum. He has an urgent CT scan which shows an acute type A aortic dissection.

What should you do next?
a. Transfer him immediately to the nearest cardiothoracic centre
b. Give titrated morphine iv for his pain
c. Start a labetalol infusion
d. Start a glyceryl trinitrate infusion
e. Give a 500-ml colloid bolus

H6

The eighth report on confidential enquiries into maternal deaths in the United Kingdom (2006–2008) was published in 2011.

Which of the following five answers has the leading causes of maternal death from that report in order of decreasing frequency (direct and indirect causes)?
a. Thrombosis/thromboembolism, sepsis, cardiac, psychiatric
b. Cardiac, other indirect causes, neurological, sepsis
c. Respiratory, diabetes mellitus, cardiac, psychiatric
d. Other indirect causes, psychiatric, anaesthesia, haemorrhage
e. Anaesthesia, pre-eclampsia/eclampsia, trauma, cardiac

H7

A 52-year-old male is on a dental list for multiple extractions. He has previously had a successful mitral valve replacement 2 years ago and is currently well. He is concerned regarding the risk of infective endocarditis associated with his surgery.

What should you inform him?
a. Antibiotic prophylaxis will be given
b. Antibiotic prophylaxis and chlorhexidine mouthwash will be given
c. Antibiotic prophylaxis is not required, but chlorhexidine mouthwash should be used

d. Neither antibiotic prophylaxis nor chlorhexidine mouthwash is required, but good oral hygiene should be maintained

e. The dental surgeons will decide if any antibiotics are necessary

H8

A healthy 25-year-old male requires an appendicectomy, with a rapid sequence induction. Following optimal preoxygenation, induction of anaesthesia and an appropriate dose of suxamethonium, your initial two attempts at intubation are unsuccessful.

The next appropriate step in your management would be:

a. Insert a laryngeal mask airway and call for help

b. Perform a fibre-optic intubation

c. Release cricoid pressure and re-attempt intubation

d. Check the position of the patients head and neck and re-attempt intubation with a McCoy (or alternative) blade

e. Place the patient in the head down, left lateral position and allow to wake whilst maintaining oxygenation

H9

The pulmonary artery flotation catheter (PAFC) is used in a variety of areas.

Its use lies in its demonstrated ability to:

a. Perform repeated measurements of haemodynamic data

b. Reduce morbidity and mortality in cardiac intensive care patients

c. Allow accurate assessment of extravascular lung water

d. Directly measure left atrial pressure

e. Estimate cardiac output in the presence of pulmonary valve disease

H10

You are asked to see a 40-year-old woman in the anaesthetic preoperative assessment clinic. She is known to suffer from myasthenia gravis and has been scheduled for a repair of a large paraumbilical hernia under general anaesthesia. You discuss your planned perioperative management with her.

Which of the following is not an indicator of a postoperative requirement for ventilation?

a. Disease duration > 6 years

b. A history of chronic respiratory disease

c. Dose requirements of pyridostigmine of 250 mg/day

d. A preoperative vital capacity of < 2.9 l

e. Grade III myasthenia gravis

H11

A 30-year-old gentleman with a BMI of 30 is listed for open appendicectomy. He denies any other significant medical co-morbidity. You decide to perform a rapid sequence induction as he is at risk of aspiration.

Which one of the following would best ensure adequacy of preoxygenation prior to induction of anaesthesia?

a. Maintenance of a patent airway with a tight-fitting mask

b. 25° head-up position
c. Preoxygenation for at least 3 minutes
d. End-tidal oxygen fraction (F_EO_2) >0.9
e. Increasing the F_iO_2 from 21% to 90%

H12

In the UK, the diagnosis of brainstem death is made following several tests, to be completed by two doctors, of at least 5 years GMC registration, on two separate occasions.

Which of the following actions does not form part of the UK Code for the diagnosis of brainstem death?
a. Exclusion of severe electrolyte derangement
b. Measurement of body temperature
c. Testing of motor or sensory function for each cranial nerve
d. Removal of mechanical ventilation for at least 5 minutes for apnoea testing
e. Time of death recorded as that at the first set of testing

H13

An 80-kg man has been involved in a fire in a first-floor flat. He has escaped by jumping out of a window. He arrives in the emergency department immobilized on a spinal board on high-flow oxygen and has had 1000 ml of 0.9% saline. He has suffered approximately 25% BSA burns. On examination: the airway is patent, but he has signs of smoke inhalation. Chest is clear bilaterally. SpO_2 98%. Blood pressure 80/35 mmHg. Heart rate 120/min. GCS 13/15 (M6 V4 E3).

What would be the most appropriate first course of action from the following?
a. Remove the cervical spine protection, get skilled assistance to perform manual in-line stabilization, perform a rapid sequence induction and secure the airway
b. Secure central venous access, and start a crystalloid infusion at 375 ml/h
c. Urgent referral to a burns unit
d. Take blood for cross-match
e. Give analgesia

H14

A 42-year-old female presents to the emergency department with a GCS 6/15. She is intubated and ventilated prior to performing a CT scan of the head. This reveals a subarachnoid haemorrhage. On transfer to ICU, the patient desaturates to 88%, despite increasing F_iO_2 of 1.0. Lung compliance is reduced and CXR reveals bilateral interstitial shadowing. ECG shows widespread T-wave inversion. Troponin I is elevated at 1.4 and echocardiogram demonstrates a mildly impaired left ventricle.

The most likely diagnosis is?
a. Adult respiratory distress syndrome
b. Acute myocardial infarction
c. Neurogenic pulmonary oedema
d. Fluid overload
e. Aspiration pneumonitis

H15

You are fast bleeped to the emergency department because there is a 1-month-old infant who has breathing difficulties. The paediatrician suspects bronchiolitis and is considering intubation and ventilation.

Which one of the following is the greatest clinical indication for intubation and ventilation?
a. Respiratory rate of 70 breaths per minute and intercostal recession
b. Respiratory rate of 70 breaths per minute, nasal flaring, heart rate of 180 per minute
c. Oxygen saturations at 88% on room air
d. Recurrent apnoeic episodes with increasing frequency
e. Inability to complete feeds due to respiratory distress

H16

A 48-year-old male with advanced HIV disease on antiretroviral therapy complains of severe burning pain and paraesthesia in the soles of his feet. On examination, ankle jerks are absent and there is blunting of sensation and vibration in both feet.

With which of the following is this best treated?
a. Duloxetine 60 mg od
b. Stopping the antiretroviral therapy
c. TENS machine
d. Oxycodone 10 mg bd
e. Pregabalin 300 mg bd

H17

You are asked to review a 25-year-old man who has been on ICU for 4 weeks with cervical cord injury (C6–7). He looks sweaty and is complaining of a headache. He has been oliguric for 2 hours but prior to that his urine output had been good. His blood pressure is 220/100 mmHg with a heart rate of 35 bpm.

What is the most likely diagnosis?
a. Malignant hypertension
b. Acute renal failure
c. Sympathetic hyper-reflexia
d. Vagal reflex
e. Raised intracranial pressure

H18

Patients with chronic liver disease will often be anaemic.

Which of the following is not a recognized cause of anaemia in patients with chronic liver disease?
a. Hypersplenism-induced haemolysis
b. Chronic illness
c. Hypoerythropoietinaemia
d. Chronic GI blood loss
e. Malnutrition

H19

You are involved in the management of a mother with a major postpartum haemorrhage (PPH), secondary to uterine atony. There are numerous pharmacological agents available to help you manage this situation.

Which of the following drug doses is incorrect?
a. Oxytocin – 5 units intravenously
b. Ergometrine 0.5 mg intravenously
c. Oxytocin infusion – 10 units/h intravenously
d. Carboprost – 250 mcg intramuscularly
e. Misoprostol – 400 mcg rectally

H20

A 2-year-old child undergoes surgery to amputate a finger following ischaemic damage from a tourniquet that was left on unnoticed. The parents consider the doctor who left the tourniquet on to be negligent. As the child grows up, he decides to sue the doctor for negligence. The child is now 14 years old.

By what age must the child start proceedings for his case to be valid?
a. He cannot because his parents should have done it within 3 years of the incident
b. 16 years old
c. 18 years old
d. 21 years old
e. There is no time limit

H21

A 50-year-old man presents to your chronic pain clinic for a review of medications. He has been using a fentanyl patch for lumbar back pain for 5 years with the current dose at 75 mcg/h, as well as pregabalin 150 mg twice daily. During the course of the interview he admits to a low libido and that it has left him feeling depressed.

What would be the next step in your management?
a. Advise his GP to start a course of sildenafil
b. Check his testosterone levels
c. Prescribe an antidepressant
d. Reduce his pregabalin to 75 mg twice daily
e. Refer him to your pain clinic psychologist

H22

Which of the following is least important in optimizing the delivery of transdermal drug preparations?
a. Molecular weight ≤500 kD
b. Lipophilic drug preparation
c. Uncharged molecule
d. Low melting point
e. Thin, well-perfused skin

H23

A 22-year-old active cross-country runner presents for an open reduction and internal fixation of a non-united ankle fracture. Despite immobilization for 8 weeks and administration of paracetamol, ibuprofen and codeine in appropriate doses, the patient complains of severe pain in the foot. The foot is cool with smooth skin and obvious allodynia and hyperalgesia.

The most appropriate anaesthetic technique for this patient is:
a. Volatile general anaesthesia with postoperative multi-modal analgesia
b. Combined femoral and sciatic block under sedation with postoperative multi-modal analgesia
c. Spinal anaesthesia with postoperative multi-modal analgesia
d. Combined spinal–epidural anaesthesia with postoperative multi-modal analgesia, including epidural local analgesia
e. Total intravenous anaesthesia (TIVA) with postoperative multi-modal analgesia

H24

A 2-year-old child is listed to have an inguinal hernia repair. You decide to perform a general anaesthetic with a caudal epidural.

Which of the following caudal epidural drugs and doses are appropriate?
a. 0.25% bupivacaine 1.5 ml/kg
b. 0.25% bupivacaine 1.0 ml/kg
c. Ketamine 1 mg/kg
d. Morphine 1 mcg/kg
e. Clonidine 10 mcg/kg

H25

A patient with an isolated head injury is brought into the emergency department. The ambulance crew state he fell from a garage roof, hitting his head. He has been unresponsive, but vomited in the ambulance on the way to hospital. His blood pressure is 160/90 mmHg, HR 90/min, S_pO_2 98% on a 15 l mask with a reservoir bag. He is on a spinal board with a cervical collar and blocks *in situ*. When the emergency department specialist registrar performs a sternal rub, the patient groans and flexes both arms. His eyes remain closed. The emergency department registrar wants to perform a CT scan of the patient's head and C-spine. The radiographer is ready and waiting.

Which of the following is the most appropriate course of action?
a. Take the patient straight to the scanner and phone the neurosurgeon to review the scans
b. Ask the emergency department nurse to accompany the patient to the scanner and to contact you again if further input is required
c. Turn the patient lateral and accompany him to the CT scanner
d. Perform a rapid sequence induction and take the patient to the scanner sedated, intubated and ventilated
e. Insert an arterial line for blood pressure monitoring before accompanying the patient to the CT scanner

H26

Which of the following respiratory pathogens has been shown to be resistant to rifampicin?

a. Panton–Valentine leukocidin-producing *Staphylococcus aureus* (PVL-SA)
b. *Legionella pneumophilia*
c. *Pseudomonas aeruginosa*
d. Methicillin-resistant *Staphylococcus aureus* (MRSA)
e. *Mycobacterium tuberculosis*

H27

A general practitioner refers an 80-year-old lady to the chronic pain clinic. The patient reports burning pain on her trunk since an episode of shingles 2 years previously. She has been on gabapentin and amitriptyline for the last 3 months with minimal improvement in her symptoms.

Which of the following would be the most appropriate next step in her management?
a. Replace the amitriptyline with venlafaxine
b. Prescribe 5% lidocaine patches
c. Prescribe transdermal fentanyl
d. Commence oral oxycodone 5 mg 6-hourly
e. Refer to a pain management programme

H28

A 57-year-old normotensive female presents with a grade-2 subarachnoid haemorrhage secondary to rupture of an anterior communicating artery aneurysm. The aneurysm is coiled uneventfully and she is admitted to the critical care unit for observation. Three days later she develops weakness in her right arm and leg. Brain computed tomography (CT) is reported as normal.

Which of the following is the most appropriate initial intervention?
a. Commencement of a nimodipine intravenous infusion at 1 mg/h and maintenance of systolic blood pressure of 180 mmHg
b. Administer titrated intra-arterial papaverine
c. Administer aspirin 300 mg and commence a heparin infusion titrated to APTT 2.5–3.0
d. Urgent catheter angiography and balloon angioplasty
e. Commencement of nimodipine 60 mg NG 4-hourly and maintenance of systolic blood pressure of 180 mmHg

H29

Paravertebral blocks can be used for both acute and chronic pain in a variety of anatomical locations.

Which of the following is most accurate?
a. Thoracic surgery is not well suited to analgesia from paravertebral blocks
b. The paravertebral space begins around T1 and finishes in the low lumbar region
c. A paravertebral injection typically blocks up to six dermatomal levels
d. The incidence of local anaesthetic toxicity is comparable to an epidural injection
e. Severe coagulopathy is a relative contra-indication

H30

A previously fit 80-kg 59-year-old Afro-Caribbean man is in hospital with an acute ascending polyneuropathy.

Which of the following observations is most sensitive predictor of need for critical care?
a. A blood pressure of 85/45 mmHg
b. A respiratory rate of 28 breaths per minute
c. A peak flow rate of 250 l/min
d. A vital capacity of 900 ml
e. A VAS pain score of 7 out of 10

Chapter 8

Paper H – Answers

H1

Answer: b.

Deep vein thrombosis and pulmonary embolus are common and potentially preventable causes of morbidity and mortality in hospital. NICE have published recently updated guidance on reducing the risk of thrombosis in patients admitted to hospital. Factors predisposing to VTE can be divided into:

- Vascular stasis/endothelial damage (immobility; indwelling lines)
- Thrombophilias (Factor V Leiden, protein C/S deficiency, lupus anticoagulant)
- Medical conditions (malignancy, congestive cardiac failure, pregnancy, inflammatory states)
- Drugs (hormonal therapies)
- Other (age, smoking status, ethnicity)

There is a very small increased risk of VTE in males (male:female ratio is 1.2:1), but other risk factors predominate.

Barker RC, Marval P. Venous thromboembolism: risks and prevention. *Contin Educ Anaesth Crit Care Pain* 2011; **11**(1): 18–23

National Institute of Clinical Excellence. Clinical guideline 92. *Venous Thromboembolism: Reducing the Risk of Venous Thromboembolism in Patients Admitted to Hospital.* 2010

H2

Answer: a.

PPH is defined as the loss of 500 ml or more of blood from the genital tract within 24 hours of the birth of a baby. It is classified into minor (500–1000 ml) and major (>1000 ml). Major PPH is subdivided into moderate (1000–2000 ml) and severe (>2000 ml). Women of Asian ethnicity have an increased risk of PPH, not Afro-Caribbean. Hypotension is detrimental in PPH; without adequate perfusion intravenous oxytocics will not reach their site of action in the uterus. A maximum of 3.5 litres of clear fluid should be administered (2 litres of warmed Hartmann's solution, followed by 1.5 litres of warmed colloid) whilst awaiting compatible blood. The oxytocin dose described is used to augment labour antenatally. Postnatally the dose usually used is 10 iu/h.

Mavrides E, Penney GC, Arulkumaran S. Prevention and Management of Postpartum Haemorrhage. Guideline London: Royal College of Obstetricians and Gynaecologists.

H3

Answer: c.

Pyloric stenosis classically presents with non-bilious, projectile vomiting in a baby boy between 3–6 weeks of age. The boy:girl ratio is about 4:1. On examination, an 'olive' mass may be palpated in the epigastrium and diagnosis is confirmed by ultrasound. Pyloric stenosis is not usually associated with other congenital abnormalities. The typical metabolic derangement is a metabolic alkalosis with hypochloraemia and hypokalaemia, which results from persistent vomiting.

Traditionally, the preferred method of induction was rapid sequence induction, but recent surveys have shown a variety of induction methods are being used. Preoperatively, the stomach should be decompressed and a nasogastric tube should provide free drainage. This can be aspirated with the patient in various positions to ensure as complete emptying of the stomach as possible before induction.

Postoperatively the baby should be closely monitored for apnoeas as these are common. It is thought that they may be partially due to disruption of cerebrospinal fluid electrolytes caused by the metabolic derangement. The baby should be monitored with pulse oximetry and apnoea monitors for the first 12–24 hours and may require supplemental oxygen.

It is also important to closely monitor blood glucose as severe hypoglycaemia may occur due to depletion of liver glycogen stores. Intravenous glucose solutions should be continued until the baby has an adequate oral intake.

Black A, McEwan A. Chapter 8: Anaesthesia for specific neonatal conditions, in *Paediatric and Neonatal Anaesthesia*, 2004. Michigan: Butterworth-Heinemann, 79–88.
Yao F, Fontes ML, Malhotra V. *Yao and Artusio's Anesthesiology: Problem-Orientated Patient Management*, 6th edn, 2008. Philidephia: Lippincott Williams & Wilkins, 514–526.

H4

Answer: d.

The surgical treatments for lung cancer include segmentectomy (where part of a single lobe is resected), lobectomy (where a single lobe is resected, either via an open or thorascopic approach – video-assisted thoracic surgery) or pneumonectomy (where an entire lung is resected).

Patients must be assessed for their suitability for surgery, with increasing amounts of resection requiring a better underlying reserve, not necessarily because the surgery is more extensive, but because as more lung is resected, less volume of healthy lung remains postoperatively.

Suitability for resection is chiefly determined by lung function tests. Predictors of suitability for a lobectomy include a preoperative FEV_1 of >1500 ml and predictors of suitability for pneumonectomy are a preoperative FEV_1 of >2000 ml.

Other indicators of suitability for pneumonectomy include a preoperative $FEV_1 > 80\%$ of predicted, a predicted postoperative $FEV_1 > 40\%$ (of preoperative FEV_1), and a maximal VO_2 of > 15 ml/kg/min. VO_2 may be determined by cardiopulmonary exercise testing when patients are unable to perform lung function tests.

Gould G, Pearce A. Assessment of suitability for lung resection. *Contin Educ Anaesth Crit Care Pain* 2006; **6**: 97–100

H5

Answer: b.

Aortic dissection is a rare but potentially fatal condition. Classification is based on the location of dissection and its duration. Stanford A dissections involve the ascending aorta, but may extend into the arch and descending aorta; these dissections usually require urgent surgery. Type B dissection involves the descending aorta only and may be managed medically under most conditions.

Clinical features include: abrupt, sharp, 'ripping' chest pain (most common in type A dissection), back or abdominal pain (more common in type B dissection). Patients may be tachycardic and hypertensive due to anxiety and pain. Later, tachycardia and hypotension may ensue from aortic rupture, pericardial tamponade, acute aortic valve regurgitation and myocardial ischaemia. Twenty per cent of patients with type A dissection have ischaemic changes on ECG due to extension of the dissection into a coronary ostium.

Aortic dissection can be easily missed and a high index of suspicion is important in patients with predisposing risk factors such as hypertension, aneurysmal disease of the aorta and connective tissue disease. The diagnosis can be made by CXR (showing widened mediastinum, haemothorax and cardiomegaly) and confirmed by either CT scan or trans-thoracic echocardiography in the unstable patient.

Initial management includes pain relief and preventing further extension of the dissection or rupture. This is achieved by using beta-blockers in the first instance (iv esmolol or metoprolol) or labetalol aiming to maintain the systolic blood pressure around 110–120 mmHg. If further reduction in blood pressure is required, then sodium nitroprusside, glyceryl trinitrate or hydralazine can be used. beta-blockers should be given before vaso-dilators, as the reflex catecholamine release due to vasodilation may increase left ventricular contraction and cause the dissection to extend. Intubation and ventilation are appropriate if there is profound haemodynamic instability or low GCS. Transfer should be arranged to a regional cardiothoracic centre as soon as possible.

Hebballi R, Swanevelder J. Diagnosis and management of aortic dissection. *Contin Educ Anaesth Crit Care Pain* 2009; **9**(1): 14–18

H6

Answer: b.

The leading causes of maternal death in the period 2006–2008 were: cardiac, other indirect causes, neurological and sepsis. There were seven anaesthetic-related deaths compared with six in each of the two previous reports.

Two of the deaths were related to a failure to oxygenate; one was following induction of general anaesthesia and the other following dislodgement of a tracheostomy tube on a critical care unit. Four women died during the postoperative period. These included complications from opiate use in a woman receiving patient-controlled analgesia, acute circulatory failure possibly secondary to a blood transfusion reaction, and a cardiac arrest during a general anaesthetic for a surgical abortion. The fourth postoperative death occurred in a woman who underwent a Category 1 section under general anaesthesia shortly after eating a meal. It was felt that she aspirated gastric contents following tracheal extubation.

The final death was caused by acute haemorrhagic-disseminated leukoencephalitis. Autopsy revealed an empyema at the lower thoracic and lumbar spinal levels and it was felt that this was the trigger, the likely causative event being the spinal anaesthetic administered for the Caesarean section.

Saving mothers' lives: Reviewing maternal deaths to make motherhood safer: 2006–2008. *Br J Obst Gynaecol* 2011; **118**: 102–108

H7

Answer: d.

This question refers to the NICE guidelines on prophylaxis against infective endocarditis. They state the following:

> Offer people at risk of infective endocarditis clear and consistent information about prevention, including:
> - The benefits and risks of antibiotic prophylaxis, and an explanation of why antibiotic prophylaxis is no longer routinely recommended
> - The importance of maintaining good oral health
> - Symptoms that may indicate infective endocarditis and when to seek expert advice
> - The risks of undergoing invasive procedures, including non-medical procedures such as body piercing or tattooing

Prophylaxis should not be offered:

- To people undergoing dental procedures
- To people undergoing non-dental procedures at the following sites: upper and lower gastrointestinal tract, genitourinary tract (this includes urological, gynaecological and obstetric procedures and childbirth), upper and lower respiratory tract (this includes ear, nose and throat procedures) and bronchoscopy.
- Do not offer chlorhexidine mouthwash as prophylaxis against infective endocarditis to people at risk undergoing dental procedures.

National Institute of Clinical Excellence. *Prophylaxis Against Infective Endocarditis*. NICE Clinical Guideline 64, 2008

H8

Answer: d.

Difficult Airway Society Guidelines 2004

Please refer to the DAS guidelines in conjunction with this explanation.

Within this scenario, Plan A would include up to three attempts at intubation, with optimization of patient position, the consideration of *reducing* cricoid pressure and the use of simple adjuncts and alternative laryngoscopes.

After three attempts, if intubation remains unsuccessful, then 'failed intubation' should be announced, and no further attempts made. In this scenario there is no Plan B, and you would move to Plan C; maintaining oxygenation whilst the patient awakens.

The DAS guidelines can be found at www.das.uk.com/guidelines/downloads.html

H9

Answer: a.

b. c. d. and e. are just wrong. There is no evidence that the use of pulmonary artery flotation catheters (PAFC) *per se* reduces morbidity and mortality. Any association between their usage and worse outcomes is confounded by the problem of selection bias – those patients most likely to benefit from invasive cardiac output and pressure monitoring are those most critically ill. EVLWI (extravascular lung water index) is used with PICC lines. Left atrial pressure is measured indirectly via wedge pressure. Pulmonary valve disease may limit the usefulness of PAFCs.

Harvey S, Young D, Brampton W *et al.* Pulmonary artery catheters for adult patients in intensive care. *Cochrane Database Syst Rev* 2006 (Online)

H10

Answer: c.

Myasthenia gravis (MG) is an autoimmune disease predominantly affecting younger women and older men. IgG antibodies attack acetylcholine receptors (AChR) at the postsynaptic membrane of the neuromuscular junction. This prevents binding of ACh to its receptor and increases AChR degradation, which results in damage to the postsynaptic membrane. The condition is associated with thymus hyperplasia in >75% of patients, as this is thought to be the site of antibody production.

Clinical features of MG include: weakness and fatigue of skeletal muscles (proximal > distal); partial and unilateral ptosis, diplopia, blurred vision; bulbar involvement; respiratory muscle involvement (20%–30%); sparing of sensory and reflex abnormalities and, finally, side effects of long-term steroid treatment. Bulbar and respiratory involvement is of particular relevance to anaesthesia.

Bulbar weakness increases risk of pulmonary aspiration, therefore patients may need RSI. MG patients may be resistant to suxamethonium. Respiratory weakness decreases clearance of secretions and therefore makes these patients prone to postoperative LRTI. Up to 30% of patients may require postoperative ventilatory support. Predictive factors include: advanced generalized disease; disease duration >6 years; concurrent chronic respiratory disease and VC <2.9 l. High-dose preoperative anticholinesterase requirements are also a risk factor. However, the dose stated above would be considered relatively modest and a pyridostigime dose of > 750 mg/day would indicate a potential need for postoperative ventilation.

The main aims of perioperative management in patients with MG are: adequate preoperative assessment, including pulmonary function testing, optimizing ongoing therapy (anticholinesterases, steroids, plasmapheresis prior to thymectomy); considering regional techniques where possible; avoiding drugs that interfere with neuromuscular transmission (patients are highly sensitive to non-depolarizing neuromuscular blocking agents and may only require 10% of normal dose); monitoring neuromuscular function and being prepared for postoperative critical care support if required. Recovery may be complicated by a myasthenic crisis, precipitated by stress, infection or underdose of anticholinesterase. Alternatively, a cholinergic crisis (manifesting as excessive muscarinic activity) may result from excessive anticholinesterase. Therefore, these drugs should be avoided wherever possible.

Marsh S, Pittard A. Neuromuscular disorders and anaesthesia. Part 2: specific neuromuscular disorders. *Contin Educ Anaesth Crit Care Pain* 2011; 11(4): 119–123

H11

Answer: a.

Patients likely to suffer early arterial desaturation during apnoea include: the critically ill, obese, obstetric and paediatric patients. During apnoea, arterial oxygen saturation remains high until almost all of the body's reserves of oxygen have been used. Pulse oximetry is therefore not a good predictor of impending hypoxia due to its response time. When hypoxia develops, oxygen saturations decreases rapidly, at a rate close to 30% min^{-1}. For severely obese patients (BMI > 40 kg m^{-2}), preoxygenation in the 25° head-up position achieves oxygen tensions >20% higher than when pre-oxygenation is applied in the supine position.

To assess the efficacy of preoxygenation one can measure the end-tidal oxygen fraction (F_EO_2), which will give an approximation of the alveolar oxygen fraction (F_AO_2). For an adult with a normal FRC and VO_2, if the F_AO_2 is >0.9 (i.e. as would be found after effective preoxygenation, the lungs would contain ~2000 ml of oxygen (i.e. 10 times VO_2). This is less effective without a patent airway when a patient is apnoeic. If no ventilation is being attempted together with 100% oxygen, there is 'apnoeic mass-movement oxygenation'. This has been shown in animal and simulated human studies to maintain oxygen saturation for up to 100 minutes. Passive diffusion of oxygen is more effective if denitrogenation of the alveoli is as complete as possible and a tight-fitting mask is used. It is important to ensure very high oxygen fraction to extend the safe duration of apnoea; increasing the oxygen fraction applied to the airway from 90% to 100% more than doubles the time to critical hypoxia with an open airway. This has a much greater effect on time to critical hypoxia than increasing the F_iO_2 applied to the airway from 21% to 90%. It cannot be assumed therefore that a patient will remain well oxygenated after a rapid sequence induction, if no active airway management is undertaken.

Sirian R, Wills J. Physiology of apnoea and the benefits of preoxygenation. *Contin Educ Anaesth Crit Care Pain* 2009; 9(4): 105–108

H12

Answer: c.

Diagnosis of brainstem death has three major components: meeting preconditions for brainstem death, excluding those conditions which may be mistaken for brainstem death and confirming lack of activity within the brainstem.

Preconditions are a deeply unconscious, apnoeic patient, with pathology known to be consistent with brainstem death.

Clinicians must exclude any reversible causes of apnoeic coma: severe disturbances in electrolytes, temperature (over 34 °C), blood-gas parameters or haemodynamic status. Consideration must be given to the prolonged effects of sedative medication, by allowing sufficient time for metabolism and excretion, or by administering specific antagonists.

The specific brainstem death tests of cranial nerves involve:

  II Direct/consensual pupillary reflexes (sensory)

 III Direct/consensual pupillary reflexes (motor) Caloric test (vestibulocochlear reflex) (motor)

 IV Caloric test (vestibulocochlear reflex) (motor)

  V Corneal brushing (sensory), supraorbital pressure (sensory)

 VI Caloric test (vestibulocochlear reflex) (motor)

VII Corneal brushing (motor), supraorbital pressure (motor)

VIII Caloric test (vestibulocochlear reflex) (sensory)

 IX Gag reflex (sensory)

  X Gag reflex (motor), cough reflex (sensory and motor)

Cranial nerves I, XI and XII are not tested.

The apnoea test involves disconnecting the patient from mechanical ventilation for five minutes, and allowing the CO_2 to rise, to assess whether ventilation is stimulated. P_aCO_2 must rise above 6.0 kPa. 100% O_2 is insufflated into the lungs during apnoea to preserve haemodynamic stability.

Oram J, Murphy P. Diagnosis of death. *Contin Educ Anaesth Crit Care Pain* 2011; **11**(3): 77–81

H13

Answer: d.

This is a difficult, but not unrealistic scenario. Burns and trauma often present together. The key concept is to decide which problem is the greatest threat to life. With this patient, the three issues are the signs of smoke inhalation, the large burn, and the shock.

The airway is patent, but it is threatened by the smoke inhalation. The patient must be observed at all times, with frequent reassessment of the airway, and should not be transferred to another unit without intubation. However, there are no immediate indications to intubate; the patient is breathing adequately, saturating well and is not comatose.

For this patient, a second bolus of 1000 ml of 0.9% saline would be appropriate due to hypotension. This would then leave 2000 ml to give over the next 3–3.5 hours (the paramedics have already given 1 litre), plus maintenance fluids, so an appropriate infusion rate would be approximately 700 ml/h; 250 ml/h would be too slow.

Blood may be lost into the chest, abdomen or pelvis, from femoral shaft fractures, or out of the body. A clear chest would not be found if there was significant haemothorax, so an alternative source must be found; spring the pelvis, look at the long bones, get a FAST scan of the abdomen, look for injuries with rapid blood loss (is there a scalp laceration?).

The airway is a concern, the burn is a concern, but the most important step is to resuscitate this patient from hypovolaemic shock. Assessing the airway and giving oxygen/fluid bolus should always be 'ticked off' at the start of any trauma scenario, but you must move on from this and prioritize your management based on treating the greatest threats to life first. In this scenario, urgent burns referral is appropriate, but this patient is too unstable for transfer and requires immediate management of his life-threatening injuries. Analgesia is also important, but again, should not be prioritized over life-saving treatments. Taking blood for cross-match is the appropriate answer from the selection as it is the only choice that acknowledges that resuscitation of hypovolaemic shock is the most important first step.

H14

Answer: c.

The most likely answer is neurogenic pulmonary oedema. Neurogenic pulmonary oedema is a well-recognized complication of subarachnoid haemorrhage. The proposed mechanism is massive sympathetic discharge resulting in peripheral vasoconstriction and re-distribution of blood to the heart and lungs. This results in hydrostatic pulmonary oedema. Myocardial dysfunction can also occur secondary to this sympathetic discharge. There may be associated ECG changes, elevated troponin levels and varying degrees of LV dysfunction seen on echocardiography.

O'Leary R, McKinlay J. Neurogenic pulmonary oedema. *Contin Educ Anaesth Crit Care Pain* 2011; **11**(3): 87–92

H15

Answer: d.

Although the other physiological parameters are abnormal, they are not sufficient to warrant intubation and ventilation of the baby at this stage. The initial treatment for bronchiolitis is oxygen, with or without CPAP. Consider intubation in any child with the following:

- Exhaustion
- Recurrent apnoeas
- Reduced conscious level
- Worsening hypoxaemia
- Worsening hypercarbia

Samuels M, Wietska S (eds.) *Advanced Paediatric Life Support, The Practical Approach*, 5th edn, 2011. London: Wiley-Blackwell.

H16

Answer: e.

This patient is suffering with an HIV-related painful peripheral neuropathy. NICE guidelines on the treatment of neuropathic pain recommend the use of pregabalin first line. Duloxetine is a selective serotonin and noradrenaline reuptake inhibitor, which is a first-line treatment for painful diabetic neuropathy only. Antiretroviral drugs have a wide range of interactions with other drugs and can in themselves cause pain. It is therefore important to be aware of the side effects of certain antiretroviral drugs and their potential interactions with antineuropathic pain drugs. Opioids can be used in neuropathic pain with moderate success, but they are not the first line. TENS machines have a place as a useful adjunct, though good-quality evidence is lacking.

NICE Clinical guideline 96. *Neuropathic Pain: The Pharmacological Management of Neuropathic Pain in Adults in Non-specialist Settings.* 2010

H17

Answer: c.

Sympathetic hyper-reflexia is a life-threatening condition triggered by somatic or visceral stimuli below the level of the injury, classically bladder or rectal distension. Sympathetic hyper-reflexia can develop suddenly and without warning. Hyper-reflexia manifests 4–6 weeks after the initial injury, once neurogenic shock has resolved. It is common in injuries above T6 and is rare in lesions below T10. The most common causes are: urinary retention, constipation, pressure sores, peptic ulcers and surgical stimulation.

Triggering stimuli generate an ascending sensory nerve impulse that stimulates the sympathetic nervous system in the spinal cord below the level of the injury. The normal descending inhibitory mechanisms generated by the vasomotor centres cannot pass below the level of the injury and sympathetic outflow continues unchecked. The clinical picture is one of malignant hypertension with reflex bradycardia. Above the level of the injury, the parasympathetic system causes headache, sweating and nasal congestion, whilst the sympathetic system predominates below the lesion with resultant skin blotching, piloerection and cool peripheries. As their blood pressure rises, patients become more restless and agitated and may become unconscious or have strokes or seizures.

Management is mainly directed at relieving the precipitating stimuli and treating the blood pressure (usually with α-blockers).

Denton M, McKinlay J. Cervical cord injury and critical care. *Contin Educ Anaesth Crit Care Pain* 2009; **9**(3): 82–86.

H18

Answer: c.

Anaemia in patients with chronic liver disease is present secondary to chronic blood loss from the GI tract, hypersplenism-induced haemolysis, chronic illness and malnutrition. EPO plasma levels are up-regulated in patients with chronic liver disease. The regulation of plasma EPO in patients with chronic liver disease is complex and multifactorial, and the degrees of anaemia, liver dysfunction, impaired pulmonary function and cytokine alterations are the major factors in regulating plasma EPO in this patient group.

Vaja R, McNicol L, Sisley I. Anaesthesia for patients with liver disease. *Contin Educ Anaesth Crit Care Pain* 2010; **10**(1): 15–19

H19

Answer: e.

Misoprostol should be 1000 mcg rectally.

Causes for PPH can be summarized as the 'Four Ts':

- Tone (abnormality of uterine contraction)
- Tissue (retained products of conception)
- Trauma (of the genital tract)
- Thrombin (abnormal coagulation)

Uterine atony is the most common cause of PPH.

When uterine atony is perceived to be a cause of the bleeding, the following mechanical and pharmacological measures should be instituted, in turn, until the bleeding stops:

- Bimanual uterine compression (rubbing up the fundus) to stimulate contractions
- Ensure the bladder is empty (Foley catheter, leave in place)
- Oxytocin 5 units by slow intravenous injection (may have one repeat dose)
- Ergometrine 0.5 mg by slow intravenous or intramuscular injection (contra-indicated in women with hypertension)
- Oxytocin infusion (40 units at 10 units/h)
- Carboprost 0.25 mg by intramuscular injection repeated at intervals of not less than 15 minutes to a maximum of eight doses (contra-indicated in women with asthma)
- Direct intramyometrial injection of carboprost 0.5 mg (contra-indicated in women with asthma), with responsibility of the administering clinician as it is not recommended for intramyometrial use
- Misoprostol 1000 µg rectally

RCOG *Prevention and Management of Postpartum Haemorrhage*. Green-top Gudeline No. 52. http://www.rcog.org.uk/womens-health/clinical-guidance/prevention-and-management-postpartum-haemorrhage-green-top-52 Accessed 20/02/2012

H20

Answer: d.

A civil procedure for negligence in England and Wales should be started within 3 years of the alleged negligence or within 3 years of the victim becoming aware of possible negligence. In minors this means the 3 years starts from the age of maturity (18 years old). Thus the child has until he is 21 years old to make the claim.

Bryden D, Storey I. Duty of care and medical negligence. *Cont Educ Anaesth Crit Care Pain* 2011; **11**: 124–127

H21

Answer: b.

It has been recognized for some time that the chronic use of opioid medications can affect hormonal and immune function. Suppression of the hypothalamic–pituitary–adrenal–gonadal axis can lead to decreases in production of testosterone, luteinizing hormone, follicle-stimulating hormone, oestrogen and cortisol. The effect is most pronounced in patients treated with intrathecal opioids.

Gonadal suppression can lead to infertility and reduced libido and male patients can benefit from testosterone replacement.

Opioids can have an effect on the immune system either through a neuroendocrine effect or by a direct action on immune cells.

Katz N, Mazer N. The impact of opioids on the endocrine system. *Clin J Pain* 2009; **25**: 170–175

H22

Answer: a.

Drug diffusion across skin and delivery to the effect-site is affected by several factors:

- Concentration difference across the membrane
- The thickness of the membrane
- Blood flow to the skin – transdermal patches work poorly in shocked patients
- The charge on the molecule – non-ionic molecules transverse more easily, but extremes of hydrophilicity or lipophilicity may hinder drug delivery
- The size of the molecule – molecules <500 D diffuse more easily (molecules as large as 500 kD will diffuse less well).
- The melting point of the drug – affects drug release.
- The potency of the drug will not alter diffusion, but will be important for drug effect. High-potency drugs such as fentanyl require relatively low doses to achieve good effect.

Bajaj S, Whiteman A, Brander B. Transdermal drug delivery in pain management. *Contin Educ Anaesth Crit Care Pain* 2011; **11**(2): 39–43

H23

Answer: d.

This patient has CRPS type 1. There is no effect of volatile or intravenous anaesthetics on outcome from CRPS. Spinal anaesthesia provides a sympathectomy essential for treatment of CRPS, but this is of limited duration. Single-shot nerve blocks provide postganglionic sympathectomy, also of limited duration. Epidural anaesthesia combined with the rapid onset of a spinal would be an ideal technique. The postoperative local anaesthetic provides a preganglionic sympathectomy that can be prolonged if pain recurs when local anaesthetic is stopped. If pain persists after 48 hours of sympathectomy, a surgical lumbar sympathectomy may be considered.

Shipton EA. Complex regional pain syndrome – mechanisms, diagnosis, and management. *Curr Anaesth Crit Care* 2009; **20**: 209–214.

H24

Answer: b.

For surgical procedures below the umbilicus caudal anaesthesia remains a popular technique of epidural blockade in children. It is performed as a single-shot technique or, occasionally, placement of epidural catheter for continuous infusion is considered.

The dosage prescription scheme of Armitage still remains the most dependable (0.25% bupivacaine):

0.5 ml/kg	All sacral dermatomes are blocked
1.0 ml/kg	All sacral and lumbar dermatomes are blocked
1.25 ml/kg	Upper limit of anaesthesia is at least mid thoracic

Note that, when 1.25 ml/kg is injected there is danger of excessive rostral spread. It is therefore considered best not to administer more that 1.0 ml/kg of local anaesthetic. Ketamine is used in caudal anaesthesia to prolong the duration of the block, but the dose given is too high. The doses d. and e. are too low.

Armitage EN. Regional anaesthesia in paediatrics. *Clin Anesthesiol* 1985; **3**: 553–558
Dalens B, Hasnaoui A. Caudal anesthesia in pediatric surgery: Success rate and adverse effects in 750 consecutive patients. *Anesth Analg* 1989; **68**: 83–89

H25

Answer: d.

From the description above, the patient has a GCS of 6/15. This means he may not be capable of protecting his airway and he has already vomited en route to the hospital. Transferring him to the scanner without intubation and ventilation puts him at high risk of aspiration. Optimal head injury management would also involve a 15-degree head up tilt and control of his P_aO_2 and P_aCO_2.

Mishra LD, Rajkumar N, Hancock SM. Current controversies in neuroanaesthesia, head injury management and neuro critical care. *Contin Educ Anaesth Crit Care Pain* 2006; 6(2): 79–82

H26

Answer: c.

Rifampicin is a bacteriocidal antibiotic drug and well established in the management of tuberculosis, where it is a first-line treatment. It may also be used to treat pneumonia caused by *L. pneumophilia. Legionella* pneumonia is often treated with a macrolide (e.g. clarithromycin) or fluoroquinolone (e.g. levofloxacin), but severe, life-threatening infections or disease in immunocompromised may be treated more effectively by combination therapy with rifampicin. The British Thoracic Society guidelines for the management of community-acquired pneumonia recommend adding in rifampicin to combination antibiotic therapy for PVL-SA and MRSA. Caution must always be exercised when administering rifampicin, due to its potential to cause both severe hepatotoxicity and drug interactions via induction of the cytochrome P450 system. *Pseudomonas aeruginosa* is resistant to rifampicin, via a number of mechanisms.

Varner TR, Bookstaver PB, Rudisill, PB. *et al.* Role of rifampin-based combination therapy for severe community-acquired *Legionella pneumophilia* pneumonia. *Ann Pharmacother.* 2011; **45**: 967–976

H27

Answer: b.

This lady is suffering from postherpetic neuralgia (PHN), a form of neuropathic pain. She is already on second-line oral treatment (tricyclic antidepressants and anticonvulsant).

Several classes of drugs are used in the treatment of PHN: topical agents, antidepressants, anticonvulsants and opioids. It is best to start with drugs that have minimal adverse effects or potentially beneficial side effects e.g. sedating TCAs in patients suffering with insomnia.

In this case the next step would traditionally be to add a strong opioid. However, newer treatments are becoming available and lidocaine in patch form has very few systemic side effects and would be worth trying first. Changing amitriptyline to venlafaxine would only be indicated if the patient was intolerant of TCAs. It may have a better effect on co-existent depression though – working via a differing mechanism.

Allen S. Pharmacotherapy of neuropathic pain. *Contin Educ Anaesth Crit Care Pain* 2005; 5(4): 134–137

Sampathkumar P, Drage LA, Martin DP. Herpes zoster (shingles) and postherpetic neuralgia. *Mayo Clin Proc* 2009; **84(3)**: 274–280

H28

Answer: e.

Subarachnoid haemorrhage (SAH) is associated with a number of neurological complications, including cerebral vasospasm, rebleeding, hydrocephalus and seizures. Angiographically demonstrable cerebral vasospasm complicates up to 70% of SAH, though fewer patients (up to 30%) present clinically. Vasospasm commonly manifests as delayed neurological deficit occurring 3–12 days after initial presentation. Neurological deficit may range from mild impairments to hemiparesis and coma.

Nimodipine is a calcium channel blocker used in the prophylaxis and treatment of vasospasm. A meta-analysis of seven trials in 1996 demonstrated an increase in odds ratio (OR) for good outcome from SAH and a decrease in OR for deficits or mortality when patients were treated with nimodipine. Enteral nimodipine 60 mg 4-hourly is a standard treatment regimen. Intravenous nimodipine can be utilized where the enteral route is not possible, but is associated with a greater incidence of hypotension.

'Triple-H' therapy (hypertension, hypervolaemia and haemodilution) is the mainstay of treatment for clinically evident vasospasm. Principal treatment targets include:

- Fluid loading to achieve a raised central venous pressure and a haematocrit of 0.3–0.35
- Vasopressors to achieve a systolic blood pressure of 160–200 mmHg (120–150 mmHg in untreated aneurysms)

Whilst there is limited evidence for its efficacy, an increase in cerebral perfusion pressure and reduction in blood viscosity clearly has the potential to reverse cerebral ischaemia. Where available, such therapy may be usefully guided by transcranial Doppler.

Balloon angioplasty may be a useful treatment for persistent neurological deficits not responding to medical therapy, though is unlikely to be the initial treatment of choice. Whilst intra-arterial papaverine may be effective in reversing angiographic vasospasm, its superiority to conventional medical treatment has not been demonstrated.

Priebe H-J. Aneurysmal subarachnoid haemorrhage and the anaesthetist. *Br J Anaesth* 2007; **99**: 102–118

H29

Answer: e.

The paravertebral space extends from T1 to T12 and is bounded by the vertebral column medially, the parietal pleura anteriorly and the thoracic transverse processes and their intervening tissue posterolaterally. The space contains the spinal nerves, grey and white rami communicantes, sympathetic chain, blood vessels and loosely connected fat. An injection at one level of 20 ml will spread to block the dermatome above and the dermatome below with a high degree of reliability. Choice of local anaesthetic concentration depends on the total number of blocks that will be required. Some authorities argue that bilateral blocks present little advantage over a thoracic epidural.

Severe coagulopathy is a relative contra-indication to paravertebral blocks. It must be borne in mind that bleeding into the intrapleural space may be copious if there are coagulation abnormalities. The risks of neural damage are significantly lower than with neuraxial blocks.

Tighe SQM, Greene MD, Rajadurai N. Paravertebral block. *Contin Educ Anaesth Crit Care Pain* 2010; **10**(5): 133–137

H30

Answer: d.

Guillain–Barré syndrome (GBS) is a progressive demyelinating disorder characterized by proximal skeletal muscle paralysis. This can be acute or subacute. Perioperative respiratory support is likely to be necessary. There is also marked autonomic dysfunction. Patients may not require any muscle relaxation. Non-depolarizing relaxants may have an exaggerated effect and should be used cautiously. Suxamethonium can cause a rapid and fatal potassium efflux and is therefore contra-indicated. Intraoperative temperature monitoring is important.

Richards KJC, Cohen AT. Guillain Barré syndrome. *Contin Educ Anaesth Crit Care Pain* 2003; **3**(2): 46–49

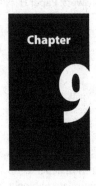

Paper J – Questions

J1

You are anaesthetizing a patient for percutaneous continuous radiofrequency (CRF) therapy for trigeminal neuralgia.

Which of the following statements is incorrect?
a. Patients are likely to be on antiepileptic medication
b. CRF therapy is a highly effective treatment for trigeminal neuralgia in the majority of patients
c. It is common for patients to be awakened during the procedure
d. CRF uses alternating current applied continuously at 100–500 Hz
e. The trigeminal ganglion is approached via the foramen ovale

J2

A 56-year-old female with a history of ischaemic heart disease presents to the pre-anaesthetic clinic for assessment prior to her thyroidectomy for multinodular goitre. She had had an NSTEMI 18 months earlier and drug-eluting stents placed in two coronary vessels, one of which is the left main stem coronary artery. She has been placed on clopidogrel and aspirin and you have been asked to consider the best course of action regarding her antiplatelet management perioperatively.

What would be your best option in her management?
a. Cease the dual platelet therapy 10 days before surgery with enoxaparin 1 mg/kg daily up to the day of surgery
b. Delay surgery for 6 months after which the clopidogrel may be ceased safely
c. Continue with the surgery as planned but ensure that platelets are administered perioperatively
d. Cease the clopidogrel, consult cardiology, consider short-acting Gp IIb/IIIa antagonist bridging therapy and continue with aspirin until the day of surgery, re-commencing clopidogrel with 600-mg loading dose on postoperative day 1
e. Cease the dual platelet therapy and admit the patient several days before surgery in order to administer a heparin infusion up until several hours preoperatively, then recommence antiplatelet therapy when confident postoperative bleeding will not be an issue

Practice Single Best Answer Questions for the Final FRCA, ed. Hozefa Ebrahim, Khalid Hasan, Mark Tindall, Michael Clarke and Natish Bindal. Published by Cambridge University Press. © Cambridge University Press 2013.

J3

A 62-year-old man presents with fever and confusion. He is agitated with a Glasgow Coma Score of 7 and is intubated in the emergency department. He has a pan systolic murmur. A transoesophageal echocardiogram reveals extensive vegetations on the native mitral valve. A Gram-positive organism is cultured from blood taken on admission.

The most likely organism is:
a. *Escherichia coli*
b. Streptococcal species
c. *Staphylococcus aureus*
d. *Pseudomonas aeruginosa*
e. Enterococci

J4

Central neuraxial blockade is used frequently in obstetric anaesthesia and analgesia. Its use is not without complications. Postpartum headache is a common occurrence.

Which of the following is most accurate?
a. Around 14% of postdural puncture headaches occur after an uneventful procedure
b. Caffeine is a proven treatment for postdural puncture headache
c. Failure of lateral eye movements is a sign of dangerous intracranial pathology
d. Most postdural puncture headaches can be treated with simple analgesia
e. Sudden onset of headache with accompanying nausea requires urgent neurological investigation

J5

A 64-year-old gentleman is admitted to the neurocritical care unit, after undergoing craniectomy for an acute right-sided subdural haematoma. Six days later his serum sodium is reported as 128 mmol/l. Serum osmolality is reduced, his central venous pressure is 1 mmHg and he has reduced skin turgor and dry mucous membranes. Urine output is 200 millilitres per hour.

Which of the following would be the most appropriate treatment for this patient's condition?
a. Demeclocycline
b. Desmopressin
c. Furosemide
d. 0.9% sodium chloride
e. Fluid restriction

J6

A 23-year-old woman attends the chronic pain clinic. She reports a 9-month history of increasing pain and immobility in her right hand. She is otherwise well, but on questioning reveals that she previously badly broke her right forearm and spent a prolonged time immobilized in a plaster cast.

From your history and examination, which of the following features is *least* important in diagnosing complex regional pain syndrome (CRPS)?
a. Positive sensory abnormalities
b. Vascular abnormalities in her right hand

c. The history of the fractured and immobilized arm
d. An absence of other conditions that could explain her pain
e. Hypohydrosis of the right arm

J7

Which of the following treatments are most useful in the treatment of life-threatening asthma?
a. Magnesium sulphate and theophylline
b. Nebulized adrenaline and continuous positive airway pressure
c. Hydrocortisone and isoflurane
d. Salbutamol and heliox
e. Ketamine and montelukast

J8

A 58-year-old man is undergoing an elective posterior fossa craniotomy in the sitting position. One hour into the operation, his SpO_2 falls from 98% to 92% and the end-tidal CO_2 level falls suddenly from 4.5 kPa to 3.1 kPa. In addition, his blood pressure drops to 70/40 mmHg from 105/65 mmHg in the absence of bleeding from the surgical field.

The first step in your immediate management plan is to:
a. Check the endotracheal tube
b. Aspirate through CVP line
c. Reduce the minute ventilation and increase FiO_2
d. Increase the PEEP to +7.5 cmH$_2$O
e. Ask the surgeon to flood the surgical site

J9

A 5-year-old, 17-kg boy with cerebral palsy develops small bowel obstruction and presents for a laparotomy. Following a rapid sequence induction using suxamethonium as the muscle relaxant, a 1.7-mg dose of vecuronium is given after 5 minutes. A second dose is required slightly sooner than expected to maintain adequate surgical conditions.

The most likely reason for this is:
a. An inadequate dose of vecuronium for the weight of the child
b. An up-regulation of acetylcholine receptors
c. Increased renal clearance
d. Incorrect drug administration
e. Patients with cerebral palsy have a relatively greater muscle mass

J10

A 26-year-old patient presents for a laparotomy for an acute abdomen. The patient informs you that she was previously addicted to heroin, but has been abstinent for 2 years. The most appropriate opioid and route to add to a multi-modal pain regime for postoperative pain management is:
a. Morphine 10 mg intramuscularly every 4 hours as needed.
b. Tramadol 20 mg every 5 minutes subcutaneously via a patient-controlled analgesia pump.

c. Pethidine 75 mg intramuscularly every 4 hours as needed.
d. Morphine 2 mg every 5 minutes subcutaneously via a patient-controlled analgesia pump.
e. Fentanyl 20 mcg every 5 minutes intravenously via a patient-controlled analgesia pump.

J11

A 30-year-old woman was admitted to the intensive care unit 24 hours ago after presenting to the emergency department following ingestion of 12 g of paracetamol approximately 24 hours before admission. She has subsequently required intubation and invasive ventilation after becoming increasingly encephalopathic. Despite supportive treatment, she has failed to improve.

Which of the following test results warrants an urgent referral to a specialist unit for consideration for liver transplantation?
a. ALT 3000 IU/l
b. Serum bilirubin 250 µmol/l
c. INR 3.0
d. Arterial lactate 3.5 mmol/l
e. Arterial pH 7.27

J12

A 75-year-old man presents for repair of an inguinal hernia. He has controlled hypertension and a history of ischaemic heart disease. He walks his dogs for 2 miles every day and can manage two flights of stairs without becoming short of breath or developing angina. He tells you he used to get exertional angina, but this has completely stopped since undergoing angioplasty 6 months ago. Looking though his notes, you see that he has a Taxus stent in his circumflex artery. The patient has had severe PONV in the past and would prefer regional anaesthesia.

What is the appropriate next step?
a. Safe to continue with general anaesthesia and surgery, but not regional anaesthesia – discuss GA with the patient, but do not agree to regional anaesthesia
b. Safe to continue with general anaesthesia and surgery, but omit clopidogrel for >10 days presurgery
c. Safe to continue with general anaesthesia and surgery, but omit aspirin and clopidogrel for >10 days presurgery
d. Delay surgery for 3 months
e. Delay surgery for 6 months

J13

In order to reduce a posterior dislocation of an ankle in a 95-kg 28-year-old rugby player, the ED registrar has asked for anaesthetic assistance as entonox is proving inadequate for the task.

The typical dose of ketamine to allow this procedure would be?
a. 9.5 ml of 100 mg/ml
b. 4.75 ml of 10 mg/ml
c. 19 ml of 10 mg/ml
d. 1.9 ml of 50 mg/ml
e. 3.8 ml of 50 mg/ml

J14

A 15-kg 3-year-old boy is scheduled for a circumcision on an elective list. He is normally fit and well. He has no known allergies and he is not on any regular medication. After induction of general anaesthesia, he receives a penile block.

Which of the following is the most appropriate additional intraoperative analgesic?
a. Paracetamol 300 mg iv, diclofenac 12.5 mg pr
b. Paracetamol 240 mg iv, diclofenac 25 mg pr
c. Paracetamol 225 mg iv, diclofenac 12.5 mg pr
d. Morphine 1.5 mg iv
e. Fentanyl 15 mcg iv

J15

A 56-year-old female presents with a 10-year history of neck pain. This pain has remained at a constant level over time and neuroimaging has not revealed any surgical pathology. There are several yellow psychosocial flags from the history.

Which would be the most appropriate tool to assess this patient's pain?
a. Visual analogue scale
b. LANSS neuropathic pain questionnaire
c. McGill pain questionnaire
d. Beck depression inventory
e. Quantitative sensory testing

J16

A 30-year-old gentleman with a BMI of 30 is listed for open appendicectomy. He denies any other significant medical co-morbidity. You decide to perform a rapid sequence induction as he is at risk of aspiration.

Which one of the following would best ensure adequacy of preoxygenation prior to induction of anaesthesia?
a. Maintenance of a patent airway with a tight-fitting mask
b. 25° head-up position
c. Preoxygenation for at least 3 minutes
d. End-tidal oxygen fraction (F_EO_2) >0.9
e. Increasing the F_iO_2 from 21% to 90%

J17

You are asked to review a 76-year-old lady in the preassessment clinic. She has a long history of bipolar disorder and refractory depression. She has been listed for a total abdominal hysterectomy. The FY1 doctor in clinic has asked for your opinion regarding her medication history and any alterations that need to be made in the perioperative period.

Which of the following psychoactive drugs would need to be stopped before surgery?
a. Lithium
b. Sodium valproate
c. Venlafaxine

d. Prochlorperazine
e. Risperidone

J18

It is recognized that volatile anaesthetic agents affect liver perfusion.

What would be the most appropriate volatile anaesthetic agent to use when anaesthetizing a patient with liver disease?
a. Halothane
b. Sevoflurane
c. Enflurane
d. Desflurane
e. Ether

J19

A 35-year-old, 26-week gestation multiparous woman presents to A&E having collapsed at home.

Which of the following is correct in the event of maternal collapse?
a. Thromboembolism is the most common cause of collapse
b. Aorto-caval compression can be significant from 26 weeks' gestation
c. Chest compressions will only achieve 30% of normal cardiac output
d. 35% of the mother's circulating volume may have already been lost prehospital
e. After 20 weeks' gestation, perimortem Caesarean section should be achieved within 4 minutes

J20

A 6-year-old boy falls off his pedal cycle and breaks his distal radius. He is brought to the hospital by his maternal grandparents. The X-ray shows that, whilst there is no neurovascular compromise, the fracture requires manipulation under a general anaesthetic. On further questioning, the boy's mother is away for the weekend and he was left in the care of his stepfather who is married to the boy's mother and has lived with the boy since he was 18 months old. The boy's mother married his birth father 10 years ago, but divorced him when the boy was 12 months old. He lives locally but only sees the boy on his birthday each year. No court orders have been issued regarding parental responsibility.

In the absence of the boy's mother, the doctor wants to obtain consent for the procedure. Who can consent?
a. The maternal grandfather
b. The maternal grandmother
c. The boy's stepfather
d. The boy's birth father
e. None of the above, the mother must return and consent herself

J21

Chronic postsurgical pain (CPSP) has become recognized as a significant cause of postoperative morbidity.

Which of the following surgical procedures is associated with the highest prevalence of postsurgical pain?
a. Caesarean section
b. Hip replacement
c. Median sternotomy
d. Thoracotomy
e. Vasectomy

J22

Recreational diving is a popular sport in the UK despite the low temperatures of our coastal waters. Divers should be well trained in how to deal with ascent from working depths, but accidents and emergencies occur and, if faced with a diving-related injury, decompression sickness may be an accompanying problem.

Which of the following is most accuarate?
a. Decompression illness is caused by nitrous oxide bubbling out of solution as divers resurface
b. Gas bubbles usually cause neurological symptoms in patients with a patent foramen ovale
c. Bubbles of gas can form on ascent from depths of 3 meters
d. Hypothermia is beneficial
e. Vomiting is more likely to be associated with carbon monoxide in diving gas than decompression sickness

J23

A 25-year-old pregnant lady in her first trimester was seen by the GP for a chancre around her genital region. Her microscopic and serological tests confirmed primary syphilis. What is her first-line therapy of choice?
a. Doxycycline 200 mg oral × 20 days
b. Ceftriaxone 500 mg im × 10 days
c. Azithromycin 2 g oral, single dose
d. Erythromycin 500 mg qds oral × 14 days
e. Benzathine penicillin G 1.8 g im single dose

J24

You are anaesthetizing a 2-year-old boy for elective bilateral inguinal hernia repair. When you turn the child onto his side in order to insert a caudal anaesthetic, you notice that he has some irregular marks on his back and buttock. You are not sure what these are.

What is the most appropriate course of action?
a. Recognize that the marks are probably normal in a mobile 2-year-old
b. Ask a senior colleague for an opinion and then contact the on-call consultant paediatrician for advice
c. Take photographs as evidence and discuss with a senior colleague after the list has finished
d. Refer to social services for further appropriate action
e. Ask the child's mother for an explanation, in the first instance

J25

Following coronary artery bypass, a 67-year-old male patient is hypotensive at 87/45 mmHg and oliguric. The patient had good left ventricular function preoperatively and weighs 90 kg. He is sedated, intubated and ventilated following the operation. He is on no cardiovascular system-supporting drugs. He has a pulmonary artery flotation catheter and measurements show the following results:

SVRI 2120   CI 1.6   SV 45   PCWP 16 cm H_2O

What would be the most appropriate treatment?
a. Noradrenaline infusion
b. Dobutamine infusion
c. Infuse 500 ml of colloid
d. Adrenaline infusion
e. Intra-aortic balloon pump

J26

Patients with cardiorespiratory disease are at an increased risk of perioperative complications. Preoperative assessment of high-risk patients to quantify risk is becoming increasingly popular.

Which one of the following is not a recognized risk prediction tool for perioperative cardiorespiratory complications?
a. Lee
b. Detsky
c. Hozefa
d. Arozullah
e. Goldman

J27

You are the obstetric anaesthetist on call and you have been asked to review a lady on the postnatal ward with a headache after an uneventful labour epidural 3 days ago. She describes the headache as frontal and worse on standing up, she feels nauseous and complains of some photophobia and neck stiffness. On examination, she is apyrexial, she has an abducens nerve palsy and her GCS is 15.

What investigation would you do next?
a. Blood pressure and urinalysis
b. Urgent CT head
c. Lumbar puncture
d. MRI
e. Blood cultures

J28

A 74-year-old male has had a CABG and mitral valve repair and has been weaned off a cardiopulmonary bypass. Bypass time was 3 hours and he received two units of packed red blood cells (PRBC) while on the pump. A thromboelastograph (TEG), activated clotting time (ACT) and arterial blood gas (ABG) have been performed postprotamine. The ACT is

195

160 seconds and the ABG is within acceptable limits with a Hb of 7.2 g/dl. The plain TEG shows an R-time of 14 min (normal 8–12) and an MA of 50 (normal 45–55). The perfusionist has used a cell-saver.

The most appropriate response is:
a. No intervention at this stage
b. Administer 50 mg protamine and re-check ACT
c. Give two units of packed red blood cells
d. Assess the patient clinically and treat accordingly
e. Administer two units of FFP and two bags of pooled platelets

J29

A patient with significant reflux disease is first on your morning list, commencing in 30 minutes. The patient does not normally take any medication for his reflux disease.

Which of the following drugs is most appropriate?
a. Lansoprazole 30 mg po on the ward
b. Metoclopramide 10 mg po on the ward
c. Ranitidine 150 mg po on the ward
d. Metoclopramide 10 mg iv once in the anaesthetic room
e. Sodium citrate 0.3 M 30 ml once in the anaesthetic room

J30

A 75-year-old man presents for an elective open abdominal aortic aneurysm (AAA) repair. Which of the following statements is most accurate?
a. Eighty-eight per cent of patients presenting for elective AAA repair also have >90% occlusion of their left anterior descending coronary artery
b. A major cause of death postoperatively is failure of the anastomosis between the descending aorta and the graft.
c. Elective AAA repair has approximately 5% mortality, but this is raised to >15% in the presence of an S3 heart sound.
d. If the patient is a smoker, then they should refrain from smoking for at least 12 days before their operation.
e. Arterial lines should be placed in the right radial artery to ensure consistent readings throughout the operation.

J1

Answer: d.

Continuous radiofrequency therapy applies high-frequency alternating current (100–500 kHz) to nerves, nerve roots or ganglia, generating heat and producing a thermal lesion. Its action is similar to that of diathermy. It is used in the chronic pain setting to produce longer-term relief from pain than local anaesthetic/steroid applications can achieve, and as an alternative to chemical lesioning (alcohol/phenol). Trigeminal neuralgia is treated with medical and surgical therapies. Of the medical treatments carbamezapine is effective in 90% of true trigeminal neuralgias, with phenytoin producing benefit in 60%. Surgical treatments include surgical decompression, an invasive posterior fossa operation and percutaneous radiofrequency ablation. Patients are anaesthetized and X-ray guidance is used to pass a needle through the foramen ovale to approximate the trigeminal ganglion. Patients are then awakened and the position of the needle is tested to reproduce pain or parasthaesia in the nerve distribution affected. When correctly placed, the patient is re-anaesthetized and a thermal lesion is created. The procedure is used where medical therapy has failed or is contra-indicated, and has a high (80%) and lasting (2–5 years) success rate. If ineffective, or short-lasting pain relief is obtained, the procedure can be repeated.

Rea W, Kapur S, Mutagi H. Radiofrequency therapies in chronic pain. *Contin Educ Anaesth Crit Care Pain* 2011; **11**(2): 35–38

J2

Answer: d.

This question is a tough one and open to some debate! The approach to perioperative management of antiplatelet therapy in patients with coronary stents needs to take into account the type of stent, duration and risks incurred by perioperative bleeding. Certainly, any patent with a DES that has been in place for less than 1 year should not have their dual platelet therapy ceased without close consultation with the patient's cardiologist. Anticoagulant therapy that is not in itself antiplatelet may not be sufficient to prevent a major adverse cardiac event perioperatively when a hypercoagulable state has been introduced. For this patient, a delay of 6 months may not be appropriate if there is any doubt about thyroid malignancy. A reasonable approach would be to continue the aspirin, cover with Gp IIb/IIIa antagonist (following cardiology input) and re-commence the clopidogrel postoperatively. The answer may well change if the DES has only been in for 6 months.

Korte W, Cattanco M, Chassot P-G *et al.* Peri-operative management of antiplatelet therapy in patients with coronary artery disease (consensus document) *Thromb Haemost* 2011; **105**(5): 743–749

J3

Answer: b.

The diagnosis of endocarditis can be somewhat challenging. Streptococcal species are responsible for over 50% of community-acquired infective endocarditis. Enterococcus, although a Gram-positive organism, only accounts for 5% of such cases. In hospitalized patients infection of intravascular lines has been proven to be a primary risk factor for *Staphylococcus aureus* endocarditis. *S. aureus* is the commonest organism causing endocarditis in intravenous drug abusers. *Pseudomonas* spp. are also seen in those abusing intravenous drugs. It tends to present acutely if involving the left side of the heart and surgery to replace the valve is often required.

Brusch JL. *Endocarditis Essentials*, 2011. Sudbury: Jones and Bartlett Learning

J4

Answer: e.

Around 40% of postdural puncture headaches (PDPH) follow seemingly uneventful epidurals. PDPH are generally evident within 72 hours of dural puncture and are thought to be caused by traction on sensitive structures within the cranial vault or due to vascular dilation. The pain is generally frontal or occipital and is worsened on coughing or straining and relieved by lying down. Some PDPH can be treated conservatively with simple analgesia, but in young parturients particularly this is often ineffective. Caffeine is thought to help but there are no well-conducted trials to back this up. It is thought by some that caffeine may lower the patient's seizure threshold. Nevertheless, some doctors advise the consumption of caffeinated drinks and in some cases relief is attributed to them. In severe cases of PDPH the abducens nerve can be affected by traction caused by movement of the intracerebral contents as the CSF pressure is lowered. This can cause failure of lateral gaze. There are many causes of headache during the puerperium. Some are potentially dangerous, and signs such as meningism, nausea and focal neurology should be met with suspicion until serious pathology can be confidently ruled out.

Sabharwal A, Stocks GM. Postpartum headache: diagnosis and management. *Contin Educ Anaesth Crit Care Pain* 2011; **11**(5): 181–185

J5

Answer: d.

This patient is most likely to be suffering from cerebral salt-wasting syndrome (CSWS). CSWS is defined as the 'renal loss of sodium during intracranial disorders leading to hyponatremia and a decrease in extracellular fluid volume'. CSWS is one of a spectrum of electrolyte disorders associated with neurological disease including the syndrome of inappropriate ADH secretion (SIADH) and diabetes insipidus (DI).

Hyponatraemia is the commonest electrolyte disorder in neurological disease. Epidemiological studies have suggested an incidence of hyponatraemia as high as 56% in patients with subarachnoid haemorrhage (SAH). SIADH is the commonest implicated cause, responsible for up to 63% of hyponatraemia in SAH, though CSWS is also important, being associated with up to 27% of such cases.

The underlying cause of CSWS has not been fully elucidated, though elevated secretion of brain natriuretic peptide (BNP) and atrial natriuretic peptide (ANP) has been implicated. The principal distinguishing characteristic between CSWS and SIADH is the presence of hypovolaemia and dehydration in CSWS, and euvolaemia or hypervolaemia in SIADH. CSWS is thus suggested by symptoms of dehydration and signs of hypovolaemia such as reduced CVP.

The mainstay of treatment for CSWS is replacement of fluid and sodium deficits by 0.9% saline. Hypertonic saline may be rarely required. Sodium correction should be achieved cautiously in order to avoid central pontine myelinolysis.

Demeclocycline, furosemide and fluid restriction would be appropriate treatments for SIADH. Desmopressin would be appropriate for diabetes insipidus, which would be characterized by elevated serum sodium and osmolality.

Cerdà-Esteve M, Cuadrado-Godia E, Chillaron JJ et al. Cerebral salt wasting syndrome: review. Europ J Intern Med 2008; 19: 249–254

J6

Answer: c.

Current diagnosis of complex regional pain syndrome is based on the International Association for the Study of Pain (IASP). Diagnosis is based on clinical examination. There is a clinical picture of sensory, motor and autonomic features.

There may be no history of an obvious noxious stimulus (5%–10%) for the development of CRPS and it is not required to make the diagnosis. It is, however, important to exclude the presence of other conditions that could explain the patient's symptoms.

Wilson JG, and Serpell MG. Complex regional pain syndrome. Contin Educ Anaesth Crit Care Pain 2007; 7(2): 51–54

J7

Answer: c.

Recommended treatments for life-threatening asthma include oxygen, nebulized or iv salbutamol, iv magnesium sulphate, iv steroid, iv adrenaline, ketamine, intermittent positive pressure ventilation (IPPV) and inhalational anaesthetic agents. Theophylline is an oral agent. Nebulized adrenaline and heliox may be useful in cases of upper airway obstruction. CPAP and leukotriene antagonists have no role in life-threatening asthma.

The British Thoracic Society guidelines for treatment of acute asthma in adults recommend supplemental oxygen, steroids, magnesium sulphate, β-agonists (inhaled, nebulized, iv) and ipratropium bromide. They state that all patients with severe or life-threatening asthma who do not respond to this therapy should be referred to intensive care.

Once in critical care, severe asthma may be further managed with adrenaline (sc, nebulized, iv), IPPV (low tidal volume, low rate, long expiratory time, and little or no PEEP) and inhalational anaesthetic agents.

British Thoracic Society Asthma Guidelines. (online). Available at: http://www.britthoracic.org. uk/Portals/0/Clinical%20Information/Asthma/Guidelines/qrg101%202011.pdf. Accessed 21.01.2012

Stanley D, Tunnicliffe W. Management of life-threatening asthma in adults. *Contin Educ Anaesth Crit Care Pain* 2008; **8**: 95–99.

J8

Answer: e.

This patient is suffering from a venous air embolism (VAE). VAEs may occur during any operative procedure in which the operative site is above the level of the right atrium and non-collapsible veins are exposed to atmospheric pressure, or when air or any other gas is introduced under pressure into a body cavity. The clinical presentation and complications depend on the volume and speed of air entry into the vein, and the filtering capacity of the lungs. A significant VAE may present with bronchospasm, cyanosis, hypoxaemia, hypercapnia, decreased $EtCO_2$, hypotension, cardiac dysrhythmias and cardiovascular collapse. In this case, the sudden drop in $EtCO_2$ reflects the decrease in venous return, rather than mechanical hyperventilation. VAE may also be diagnosed by the presence of a millwheel murmur using a precordial stethoscope (late sign) or a transoesophageal stethoscope.

Management of clinical venous air embolism includes measures to prevent expansion of the embolus and further entrainment of air into the venous system. Therefore, the surgeon should be notified immediately and the surgical field should be flooded with saline whilst haemostasis is obtained. F_iO_2 should be increased to 1.0. The operative site should be lowered below the level of the heart if possible. Nitrous oxide should be discontinued, as this will cause expansion of the air bubbles. If a large amount of air is entrained, and if the surgical condition permits, the left lateral decubitus (Durant) position may improve right ventricular outflow, reduce the volume of air ejected into the pulmonary circulation and allow air to accumulate within the apex of the right ventricle. This permits aspiration of air via an appropriately positioned central venous catheter, from the right side of the heart. However, this would not be the first step in your management. Blood pressure should be supported using intravenous fluids and vasopressors.

The addition of PEEP to ventilator settings can increase venous pressure and reduce entrainment of air into the venous circulation.

Mirski MA, Lele AV, Fitzsimmons L, Toung TJ. Diagnosis and treatment of vascular air embolism. *Anaesthesiology* 2007; **106**: 164–177.

J9

Answer: b.

Although it may be counter-intuitive, non-depolarizing muscle relaxants are less potent in patients with cerebral palsy. This is due to up-regulation of acetylcholine receptors; however, this may be offset clinically if the child is relatively dehydrated, as the total volume of distribution will be less. Patients with cerebral palsy tend to have atrophic muscles.

Prosser DP, Sharma N. Cerebral palsy and anaesthesia. *Contin Educ Anaesth Crit Care Pain* 2010; **10**(3): 72–76

J10

Answer: b.

The intramuscular route and as-needed mode of administration are inappropriate for acute pain management, particularly in this patient. Tramadol is the most appropriate drug for this patient, but dose requirement and pain control should be carefully monitored as escalation to morphine or fentanyl may be required, but these would not be first-line options.

Mehta V, Langford RM. Acute pain management for opioid dependent patients. *Anaesthesia* 2006; **61**: 269–276

J11

Answer: e.

Paracetamol is the commonest drug taken in overdose in the UK and knowledge of its management is extremely important, given the seriousness of the consequences. Ingestion of 12 g of paracetamol, regardless of the patient's weight, is a potentially lethal dose and in this situation, the presentation has been delayed (which is an additional risk factor). Commonly, patients are asymptomatic for the first 24 hours or have non-specific symptoms such as nausea, vomiting and abdominal pain. After this time, hepatic necrosis begins to develop due to the accumulation of the toxic metabolite, NAPQI (N-acetyl-p-benzoquinone imine). The hepatocytes in Zone 3 are particularly prone to damage in paracetamol overdose, as this is the area of the liver that is relatively poorly perfused, i.e. furthest away from the hepatic artery.

The need for liver transplant can be assessed using the King's College Criteria. These were devised in 1989 to determine if there any indices of poor prognosis with acute liver failure (ALF), and further stratified into paracetamol and non-paracetamol causes. The criteria for transplant in this situation are as follows:

- Arterial pH <7.3
- **All three** of: an INR >6.5 (PT >100s), serum creatinine >300 μmol/l and the presence of Grade III/IV encephalopathy

The LFTs themselves do not form part of the criteria in paracetamol overdose, but may have predictive value in ALF due to other causes. The King's College Criteria are instrumental in selecting patients who have a high risk of mortality with ALF and are more specific in patients with paracetamol-induced ALF. However, they have limitations, and absolute reliance upon prognostic scoring systems is not recommended.

O'Grady JG, Alexander GJ, Hayllar KM, Williams R. Early indicators of prognosis in fulminant hepatic failure. *Gastroenterology* 1989; **97**(2): 439–445.

Devlin J, O'Grady JG. Indications for referral and assessment in adult liver transplantation: a clinical guideline. *Gut* 1999; **45**: VI1–VI22

J12

Answer: e.

Coronary artery stenting is a common treatment for ischaemic heart disease, and is performed more often than coronary artery bypass grafting. Stenting is the most common form of percutaneous coronary intervention (PCI). Following balloon angio-plasty of a stenosed vessel, a metal coil (stent) is left in the artery to maintain patency. This may be a bare metal stent (BMS) or drug-eluting stent (DES). DESs contain a drug that inhibits proliferation of the coronary vascular endothelium, thereby reducing the rate and incidence of restenosis within the stent. Stents are a potential source of thrombus formation, so patients with any form of stent *in situ* are placed on dual antiplatelet therapy – often aspirin and clopidogrel. All patients require lifelong aspirin. Those with BMSs usually take clopidogrel for 6 weeks. Those with DESs usually take clopidogrel for 1 year.

There are two main concerns with surgery during the period of dual antiplatelet therapy; bleeding, and the risk of coronary thrombus formation, resulting from the proinflammatory response. However, stopping clopidogrel during the recommended treatment period can cause a 30-fold increase in stent thrombosis. Therefore, all elective non-cardiac surgery should be avoided for at least 6 weeks following insertion of a BMS and at least 1 year following insertion of a DES. For emergency, life- and limb-saving surgery within these timeframes, the effects of aspirin and clopidogrel can be reversed by platelet transfusion. For urgent surgery, e.g. cancer surgery within these timeframes, the position is difficult, and requires discussions between surgery, anaes-thesia, cardiology and critical care. The risks of stopping and not stopping antiplatelet therapy must be considered. This will depend on the site of the proposed surgery (e.g. bleeding may be more catastrophic following neurosurgery than intra-abdominal surgery), and the position of the stent (e.g. restenosis may be more or less catastrophic, depending on the anatomical position of the stent).

DeVile MP, Foex P. Anti-platelet drugs, coronary stents and non-cardiac surgery. *Contin Educ Anaesth Crit Care Pain* 2010; **10**: 187–191

J13

Answer: b.

Ketamine is a dissociative anaesthetic with a wide therapeutic index. Procedural analgesia with ketamine requires a dose of approximately 0.5 mg/kg. This means a dose of 47.5 mg in this particular patient. Therefore, only b. is correct. Larger doses of 1 mg/kg may allow considerable interventions, including prehospital surgical procedures such as thoracostomy. Further increasing the dose to 2 mg/kg will cause induction of general anaesthesia. This wide therapeutic index, along with preservation of airway reflexes, cardiac output and systemic vascular resistance makes it very suitable for use beyond theatres. It is presented in one of three concentrations and great care must be taken to ensure the correct strength is being used.

Wyatt J, Illingworth R, Robertson C. *Oxford Handbook of Emergency Medicine*, 2005. Oxford: Oxford University Press

J14

Answer: c.

The dosage for paracetamol is 15 mg/kg iv, 20 mg/kg pr, and diclofenac 1 mg/kg.

The benefits of an effective penile block would remove the need for opioids. The child is unlikely to require an overnight stay, and therefore opioids (with their associated side effects) are unnecessary. Paracetamol and NSAIDs should suffice, but the dosing of these drugs in paediatric practice should be calculated carefully.

Gandhi M and Vashisht R. Anaesthesia for paediatric urology. *Contin Educ Anaesth Crit Care Pain* 2010; **10**(5): 152–157

J15

Answer: c.

Chronic pain comprises not only physiological factors but also emotional, psychosocial and cultural factors. In the chronic pain setting, a biopsychosocial model of assessing pain is advocated. Red flags represent organic pathology, whilst yellow flags represent psychosocial barriers to recovery. These include hurt/harm beliefs, fear avoidance and depression which can exacerbate the pain problem. Narrow unidimensional measures of pain are of limited value in the chronic pain setting. The McGill pain questionnaire takes a qualitative approach to pain and gives the clinician a broader picture of the factors contributing to the patient's pain problem (i.e. sensory, affective and evaluative). The other pain measurement tools listed would be useful in combination, but in isolation are too narrow to gain a global impression of the patient's pain problem.

Melzack R. The McGill Pain Questionnaire: major properties and scoring methods. *Pain* 1975; **3**: 277–299

Holdcroft A, Jaggar S. Principles of pain evaluation in *Core Topics in Pain*, 1st edn, 2005. Cambridge University Press, 81–84

J16

Answer: a.

Patients likely to suffer early arterial desaturation during apnoea include: the critically ill, obese, obstetric and paediatric patients. During apnoea, arterial oxygen saturation remains high until almost all of the body's reserves of oxygen have been used. Pulse oximetry is therefore not a good predictor of impending hypoxia due to its response time. When hypoxia develops, oxygen saturations decreases rapidly, at a rate close to 30% min^{-1}. For severely obese patients (BMI > 40 kg m^{-2}) preoxygenation in the 25° head-up position achieves oxygen tensions >20% higher than when preoxygenation is applied in the supine position.

To assess the efficacy of preoxygenation one can measure the end-tidal oxygen fraction (F_EO_2), which will give an approximation of the alveolar oxygen fraction (F_AO_2). For an adult with a normal FRC and VO_2, if the F_AO_2 is >0.9 (i.e. as would be found after effective preoxygenation, the lungs would contain ~2000 ml of oxygen (i.e. 10 times VO_2). This is less effective without a patent airway when a patient is apnoeic. If no ventilation is being attempted together with 100% oxygen, there is 'apnoeic mass-movement oxygenation'.

This has been shown in animal and simulated human studies to maintain oxygen saturation for up to 100 minutes. Passive diffusion of oxygen is more effective if denitrogenation of the alveoli is as complete as possible and a tight-fitting mask is used. It is important to ensure very high oxygen fraction to extend the safe duration of apnoea; increasing the oxygen fraction applied to the airway from 90% to 100% more than doubles the time to critical hypoxia with an open airway. This has a much greater effect on time to critical hypoxia than increasing the F_iO_2 applied to the airway from 21% to 90%. It cannot be assumed therefore that a patient will remain well oxygenated after a rapid sequence induction, if no active airway management is undertaken.

Sirian R Wills J. Physiology of apnoea and the benefits of preoxygenation. *Contin Educ Anaesth Crit Care Pain* 2009; **9**(4): 105–108

J17

Answer: a.

Selective serotonin reuptake inhibitors (SSRIs) have become the most commonly used drugs in the treatment of depression. Interactions with certain anaesthetic agents may precipitate the serotonin syndrome (hyper-reflexia, agitation and hyperthermia). There is an increased risk of bleeding in patients taking non-steroidal anti-inflammatory drugs (NSAIDs) with an SSRI due to their interference with platelet function. Withdrawal of SSRIs may cause dizziness, gastrointestinal upset, and a variety of psychiatric symptoms. As the risks associated with remaining on an SSRI are relatively low, it is generally considered acceptable to continue them throughout the perioperative period.

Although more commonly used in the treatment of epilepsy, sodium valproate can also be used as a mood stabilizer. This is not first-line therapy, which may indicate resistant illness and increased potential for recurrence should medication be stopped.

Antipsychotics are conventionally classified as typical or atypical. Patients taking these have a high relapse rate when their medication is discontinued. A rare but significant side effect of both the typical and the atypical antipsychotic drugs is the neuroleptic malignant syndrome (hyperthermia, autonomic dysfunction and muscle rigidity) which carries 20%–30% mortality. Perioperatively, the differential diagnosis would include malignant hyperthermia.The antiadrenergic and anticholinergic effects of typical antipsychotics are unpredictable, therefore other drugs with similar effects should be used with care. It is also advisable to avoid other drugs with an antidopaminergic effect, as this action may be enhanced.

Lithium is used in the treatment of mania, bipolar disorders, and as an adjuvant for refractory depression. It has a narrow therapeutic ratio and is excreted solely by the kidneys. Lithium causes a reduction in the release of neurotransmitters in both the CNS and PNS and therefore prolongs depolarizing neuromuscular block and reduces the requirements of anaesthetic agents. NSAIDs reduce the excretion of lithium by the kidneys and can result in toxic plasma levels (>1.5 mmol/l). It is prudent that lithium is stopped at least 24 h before surgery.

Peck T, Wong A, Norman E. Anaesthetic implications of psychoactive drugs. *Contin Educ Anaesth Crit Care Pain* 2009; **9**(4): 177–181

J18

Answer: d.

All volatile agents reduce CO and MAP and therefore reduce liver blood flow. Isoflurane, sevoflurane and desflurane undergo minimal hepatic metabolism and can be regarded as safe. Desflurane is probably ideal as it is least metabolized and has the lowest blood:gas partition coefficient. It provides quickest emergence. It also relatively preserves hepatic blood flow and CO (minimal effects on hepatic arterial buffer response).

Vaja R, McNicol L, Sisley I. Anaesthesia for patients with liver disease. *Contin Educ Anaesth Crit Care Pain* 2010; **10**(1): 15–19

J19

Answer: d.

Haemorrhage is the most common cause of maternal collapse. Thromboembolism was the most common cause of maternal death in the 2003–2005 CEMACH report, although it has been superseded by sepsis and pre-eclampsia/eclampsia in the 2006–2008 report. Aortocaval compression must be considered from 20 weeks of gestation, Resuscitation Council guidelines mandate a left lateral tilt of 15°. Chest compressions in non-pregnant women will achieve around 30% of normal cardiac output at best. In pregnant women, aortocaval compression further reduces cardiac output to around 10%. Otherwise healthy pregnant women can lose up to 35% of their circulating volume before becoming symptomatic. If there is no response to CPR within 4 minutes of maternal collapse, delivery should be undertaken and should be achieved within 5 minutes.

Johnston TA, Grady K. *Maternal Collapse in Pregnancy and the Puerperium*, 2011. London: Royal College of Obstetricians and Gynaecologists

J20

Answer: d.

Consent can only be granted by someone with parental responsibility. Grandparents only have parental responsibility if issued by a court order. Since 1 December 2003 in England and Wales, unmarried fathers have parental responsibility, provided they are named on the birth certificate. If the child was born before this date or if the father is not named on the birth certificate, an unmarried father has no parental responsibility. Fathers who are married to the mother at the time of birth have parental responsibility, which doesn't change with divorce, regardless of residency of the child. Step-parents must apply for a court order to have parental responsibility. Mothers always have parental responsibility.

Williams CA, Perkins R. Consent issues for children: a law unto themselves? *Cont Educ Anaesth Crit Care Pain* 2011; **11**: 99–103

J21

Answer: d.

Although there is no official definition for chronic postsurgical pain (CPSP), the following criteria are generally used:

- Pain developing after a surgical procedure
- Pain of at least 2 months' duration
- Other causes of pain excluded, e.g. infection
- The possibility that the pain is continuing from a pre-existing pain problem must be explored and exclusion attempted

CPSP is associated with increased healthcare utilization and has a significant effect on the patient's quality of life.

The following procedures are associated with the highest prevalence of CPSP:

• Amputation	62%–70%
• Thoracotomy	50%
• Mastectomy	30%–50%
• Sternotomy	30%
• Inguinal hernia repair	23%
• Laparoscopic cholecystectomy	12%

The relationship between surgical nerve damage and the development of CPSP is not straightforward – not all patients with nerve damage will develop CPSP and patients complaining of CPSP will not always describe neuropathic pain.

There have been a number of risk factors associated with the development of CPSP; some are surgery specific, while others are more general:

- Surgical nerve injury
- Continued inflammatory response (e.g. mesh hernia repair)
- Pre-existing pain
- Severity of postoperative pain
- Radiation or chemotherapy postoperatively
- Psychological vulnerability
- Female gender
- Younger age

Strategies for preventing CPSP have shown mixed results, but reduced incidences of CPSP following mastectomy have been shown with paravertebral blockade commenced before incision and continued postoperatively. Likewise, the use of epidural analgesia for posterolateral thoracotomy. Further work is needed to examine the perioperative use of adjuvants such as gabapentin.

Searle RD, Simpson KH. Chronic post-surgical pain. *Cont Educ Anaesth Crit Care Pain* 2011: **10**(1); 12–14.

Perkins F, Ballantyne J. Postsurgical pain syndromes, in Stannard C, Kalso E, Ballantyne J. (eds.) *Evidence-based Chronic Pain Management*, 2010. Blackwell Publishing

J22

Answer: c.

The 'bends' are caused by nitrogen, which is relatively insoluble, forming bubbles as it comes out of solution during the pressure drop on ascent from a dive. There is no appreciable quantity of nitrous oxide in divers' breathing air which is simply compressed atmospheric air. Other mixtures are used in specialist applications, but none contains nitrous oxide.

There are several symptoms of decompression sickness. 'The bends' refers to pain in joints. 'The staggers' refers to neurological symptoms. 'The creeps' and 'the chokes' refer to skin and pulmonary manifestations. Neurological symptoms can occur with or without a patent foramen ovale, since nitrogen is present in arterial blood as well as venous.

Bubbles of gas have been shown to occur on ascent from depths of as little as 3 m. These bubbles are very small and are usually filtered out as blood flows through the lungs. Patients with patent foramen ovale may be at risk of paradoxical gas emboli.

Hypothermia is a significant problem in patients with decompression sickness. It contributes to cardiovascular instability. Patients should be warmed passively and should be transported horizontal to mitigate these effects.

Vomiting is a symptom of decompression sickness. It is possible, but extremely unlikely, that breathing air could be contaminated with carbon monoxide (CO). The first symptom of CO poisoning is usually headache and the first sign is a cherry red complexion of the face. CO poisoning requires treatment with oxygen at high concentration. CO poisoning can be treated with hyperbaric oxygen, but this is generally not necessary.

Pitkin AD. Hyperbaric oxygen therapy. *Contin Educ Anaesth Crit Care Pain* 2001; **1**(5): 150–156

Williams DJ. Bubble trouble: an introduction to diving medicine. *Contin Educ Anaesth Crit Care Pain* 2002; **2**(5): 144–147

J23

Answer: e.

Penicillin is the drug of choice for treating all stages of syphilis. Parenteral rather than oral treatment has been the route of choice, as the therapy is supervised and bioavailability is guaranteed. Alternative regimes are (1) amoxycillin 500 mg oral qds plus probenecid 500 mg oral qds × 14 days, (2) ceftriaxone 500 mg im × 10 days, (3) erythromycin 500 mg oral qds × 14 days, or azithromycin 500 mg oral × 10 days plus evaluation and treatment of neonates at birth with penicillin. Patients with penicillin allergy are treated with erythromycin or azithromycin, and after delivery and breast-feeding they should be treated with doxycycline.

Oswal S, Lyons G. Syphilis in pregnancy. *Contin Educ Anaesth Crit Care Pain* 2008; **8**(6): 224–227

J24

Answer: b.

The anaesthetist may encounter abused children in a number of settings, such as reviewing a sick child in A&E, having a child disclose abuse to them or as an incidental finding under anaesthesia, among others. Suspicious signs include excessive bruising (particularly in a non-ambulant child), burns or bite marks, injuries in unusual or inaccessible places and trauma without adequate history.

The safety of the child takes precedence over other duties and no concerns should be ignored. As a junior anaesthetist, it is appropriate to seek advice from a consultant and after consideration the duty paediatrician or the Trust-named Child Protection Lead should be contacted. They may not be able to attend the case immediately and it should be noted that anaesthesia should not be unreasonably prolonged in that case. If there are very serious concerns, Social Services will be informed and the responsibility for this lies with the named/ designated doctor or nurse.

Further management involves discussion with the parents or carers, further assessment (such as photography) and involving Social Services or the police. The parents may offer a reasonable explanation and, if there is uncertainty, a second opinion may be sought. The parents should be informed of this. This discussion should be lead by the Child Protection Lead Consultant and the consultant anaesthetist. Formal review and Child Protection examination requires parental consent, which should be taken by the doctor/nurse performing the examination. Photography requires consent, and photographs must not be taken in theatre without it.

All concerns and examination findings must be accurately documented. With regard to confidentiality and disclosure, doctors must disclose information about the child if they believe it to be in the child's best interests and this information may be passed on to an appropriate responsible person or a statutory agency.

Royal College of Paediatrics and Child Health. *Child Protection and the Anaesthetist: Safeguarding Children in the Operating Theatre.* Intercollegiate Document, March 2007

J25

Answer: b.

The results of the cardiac output study indicate that the cardiac index of this patient is not adequate. As

$$MABP = Cardiac\ output\ x\ SVR$$

the low cardiac index is the major determinant of this patient's hypotension. Cardiac output is the product of heart rate and stroke volume, with the later being determined by preload, contractility and after load. The PCWP is 16, which suggests that the patient's filling pressure is within normal range and so infusion of 500 ml of colloid is unlikely to be of benefit. In the above scenario improvement in the cardiac contractility is needed along with afterload reduction, making the use of dobutamine the most sensible choice.

Millers RD. Cardiac physiology, in *Miller's Anaesthesia*, 2010. Philadelphia: Churchill Livingstone.

J26

Answer: c.

Goldman, Detsky and Lee produced scoring systems to predict likelihood of cardiac complications. Arozullah produced a risk prediction equation for postoperative respiratory failure.

Goldman – This is a multi-factorial index of cardiac risk in the non-cardiac surgical setting. It was developed for preoperative identification of patients at risk from major perioperative cardiovascular complications. The data were derived retrospectively in 1977 from 1001 patients undergoing non-cardiac surgery.

Detsky – a multi-factorial cardiac risk index that can be used to assess patients undergoing non-cardiac surgery. The index is a modified version of an index that was previously generated by Goldman.

Lee – In stable patients undergoing non-urgent major non-cardiac surgery, this index can identify patients at higher risk for complications. This index may be useful for identification of candidates for further risk stratification with non-invasive technologies or other management strategies, as well as low-risk patients in whom additional evaluation is unlikely to be helpful.

Arozullah – The respiratory failure risk index is a validated model for identifying patients at risk of developing postoperative respiratory failure and may be useful for guiding perioperative respiratory care.

Agnew N. Preoperative cardiopulmonary exercise testing. *Contin Educ Anaesth Crit Care Pain* 2010; **10**(2), 33–37

J27

Answer: a.

Postpartum headache is a common symptom. Thirty-nine per cent of parturients experience headache in the first postpartum week. It is not uncommon for the obstetric anaesthetist to be asked to review women with postpartum headaches because of increasing awareness of postdural puncture headaches (PDPH) after regional anaesthesia. It is therefore essential that anaesthetists know the differential diagnosis of postpartum headache and know how to manage a patient with a suspected PDPH.

The differential diagnosis of postpartum headache includes: tension headache, migraine, pre-eclampsia/eclampsia, postdural puncture headache, cortical vein thrombosis, subarachnoid haemorrhage, posterior reversible leukoencephalopathy syndrome, space-occupying lesion, sinusitis and meningitis.

Assessment should include a thorough history, physical examination and measurement of temperature, blood pressure and urinalysis as a minimum. Between 11% and 44% of all eclamptic seizures present in the postpartum period and headache and visual disturbance might be the first warning symptoms. Blood cultures would only be indicated in the presence of fever.

Sabharwal A, Stocks GM. Postpartum headache: diagnosis and management. *Contin Educ Anaesth Crit Care Pain* 2011; **11**(5): 181–185

J28

Answer: b.

This question tests a candidate's understanding of coagulopathy; the context of cardiac surgery is secondary. A solid grasp of the traditional intrinsic–extrinsic pathways of coagulation, as well as an understanding of thromboelastography is essential for an anaesthetist involved in major surgery. The ACT is too high and requires treatment. The standard dose for protamine is often quoted as 1 mg for every 100 units of heparin administered. Due to individual variation, a repeat ACT is checked 10 minutes after protamine administration, and further protamine given if required. The plain TEG R-time is prolonged suggesting FFP may be required; however, there is no heparinase specimen and the TEG may normalize with administration of protamine. PRBCs are not indicated (yet) and to 'assess clinically and treat accordingly' is too vague a plan.

Kaplan JA ed. *Essentials of Cardiac Anesthesia* 2008. Philadelphia: Saunders

J29

Answer: e.

Oral sodium citrate solution is the only agent that will affect the pH of the fluid in the stomach at the time of administration. An oral H_2 receptor antagonist should be administered 1–2 hours in advance and a proton pump inhibitor 12 hours in advance to have any effect. They will only affect the pH of new gastric acid being produced. Metoclopramide is a prokinetic with little evidence for its use in this role.

King W. Pulmonary aspiration of gastric contents. *Update Anaesth* 2010; 5:26: 28–31.

J30

Answer: c.

Patients presenting for elective AAA repair are often in their 50s or older. They frequently have significant co-morbidities including coronary artery disease in 25%–65%. Those with diabetes mellitus, hypertension and hyperlipidaemias and smoking are at increased risk of aortic aneurysm. Patients are generally quoted a mortality of about 5% during the consent process. This mortality rises to around 20% in the presence of heart failure. The major cause of death in patients post AAA repair is myocardial infarction. Primary graft failure is very uncommon after AAA repair. Long-term graft patency has been quoted at around 95% in some studies. The major causes of primary failure are structural defects in the graft itself. Defects of various types have been reported in all available graft types.

Secondary graft failure is associated with (i.e. caused by) downstream obstruction of the vascular tree. Patients with peripheral vascular disease who have had bypass surgery for occlusive disease are at greater risk than those who have had aneurysm repair, but the association between outflow obstruction and graft failure also holds for AAA repair and places smokers at higher risk of graft failure in the long term. Infection is a potentially serious problem and carries a high risk of morbidity and mortality. Less than 2% of grafts become infected, but mortality can be as high as 50% once infection is evident.

Patients who smoke have more reactive airways than those who do not. They also produce greater volumes of pulmonary secretions perioperatively. They are more difficult to oxygenate and ventilate due to lung damage sustained through smoking and are far more likely to have co-morbid ischaemic heart disease. Postoperatively it is very important to encourage deep breathing and coughing, as they are more likely to suffer pulmonary infections. Smoking cessation should be discussed well in advance of the operation. If long-term cessation is not possible (long term being 3–4 months), then it may be better to abandon the attempt as short-term (1–4 weeks) is associated with increased secretions and therefore an increased risk of infection. Cessation for 6–48 hours reduces airway reactivity and also has beneficial effects on myocardial oxygen supply/demand.

Hope G, Wolfson S, Sutton-Tyrrell K *et al*. Risk factors for abdominal aneurysms in older adults enrolled in the Cardiovascular Health Study. *Arterioscler Thromb Vasc Biol* 1996; **16**: 963

Paper K – Questions

K1

You are asked to review a 56-year-old gentleman in the preassessment clinic. Eight months ago he suffered an acute anterior myocardial infarction and underwent primary percutaneous coronary intervention and insertion of a drug-eluting stent. He is currently taking aspirin and clopidogrel 75 mg once daily. He has been listed for removal of a blocked ureteric stent at the earliest opportunity. The FY1 doctor in clinic has asked for your opinion regarding his antiplatelet therapy in the perioperative period.

Which of the following would be the most appropriate management plan in this case?
a. Stop both aspirin and clopidogrel 5 days preoperatively
b. Continue aspirin and stop clopidogrel 5 days preoperatively
c. Continue both aspirin and clopidogrel
d. Continue aspirin, stop clopidogrel 5 days preoperatively and start low molecular weight heparin 4 days preoperatively
e. Stop aspirin and clopidogrel and start low molecular weight heparin 4 days preoperatively

K2

A 25-year-old female presents to the emergency department 30 minutes after the deliberate ingestion of 50 g paracetamol. She has a Glasgow Coma Score (GCS) of 15 and there is no evidence of cardiorespiratory compromise.

What would be the most appropriate initial treatment?
a. Gastric lavage
b. Forced alkaline diuresis
c. Induced emesis with ipecac
d. Oral administration of 50 g of activated charcoal
e. Intravenous N-acetylcysteine

K3

A 45-year-old man has been removed from a furniture warehouse fire with signs of smoke inhalation and superficial burns to his legs. On arrival in the emergency department, he is breathless and drowsy. Initial arterial blood gas analysis demonstrates a profound metabolic acidosis with measured carbon monoxide levels of 12%.

Practice Single Best Answer Questions for the Final FRCA, ed. Hozefa Ebrahim, Khalid Hasan, Mark Tindall, Michael Clarke and Natish Bindal. Published by Cambridge University Press. © Cambridge University Press 2013.

Which of the following diagnoses and treatments is most appropriate?
a. Acute alcohol intoxication – gastric lavage
b. Carbon monoxide poisoning – hyperbaric therapy
c. Hypovolaemic shock – fluid resuscitation
d. Cyanide poisoning – 100% oxygen
e. Intracerebral event – rapid CT

K4

A 25-year-old man requires surgery to suture multiple lacerations to his arm. Due to his extreme fear of general anaesthesia, he wants the procedure done while awake. The anaesthetist agrees to do this with a brachial plexus block using the interscalene approach. During the procedure the patient complains of pain.

This is likely to be in which nerve distribution?
a. Median nerve
b. Radial nerve
c. Ulnar nerve
d. Superior lateral cutaneous nerve of the arm
e. Inferior lateral cutaneous nerve of the arm

K5

A 58-year-old man with pancreatic carcinoma has persistent abdominal pain despite several attempts at optimizing analgesia. Following discussion with the patient, it is decided to perform a coeliac plexus block.

Which is the most appropriate and effective agent to use to perform the block in these circumstances?
a. 6.6% phenol
b. 0.75% ropivacaine with triamcinolone 40 mg
c. 0.5% bupivacaine with triamcinolone 40 mg
d. 15% alcohol
e. 2% lidocaine with triamcinolone 40 mg

K6

You have been asked to review a patient in the emergency department. You are handed an arterial blood gas result. Biochemical analysis shows a combination of hyperkalaemia and a metabolic acidosis with a raised anion gap.

The most likely cause is:
a. Chronic renal failure
b. Conn's disease
c. Analgesic nephropathy secondary to codeine
d. Type 1 renal tubular acidosis
e. Type 4 renal tubular acidosis

K7

A 3-year-old child (15 kg) has been listed for a procedure under general anaesthesia. The child is extremely anxious and has previously been uncooperative.

213

The most appropriate sedative premedication would be:
a. Trimeprazine 15 mg po
b. Ketamine 75 mg po
c. Midazolam 5.0 mg po
d. Midazolam 3 mg intranasal
e. Midazolam 1 mg iv

K8

A 38-year-old female is presented for an epidural steroid injection. During her preoperative evaluation she is found to have a BMI of 43 and is confirmed to have had difficult epidurals with inadequate analgesia during normal vaginal delivery of her children, the last 3 years ago.

The most useful adjunct to performing an epidural in this patient is:
a. Ultrasound
b. Preoperative CT scan
c. Fluoroscopy screening
d. Peripheral nerve stimulation
e. An extra-long epidural needle

K9

Delirium on the intensive care unit is a very common issue. You are asked to see a 78-year-old man who is confused and agitated following an emergency abdominal aortic aneurysm repair.

Which of the following is the most sensitive and appropriate tool for assessing and diagnosing delirium in a ventilated patient?
a. RASS
b. Ramsay Scale
c. ICDSC
d. CAM-ICU
e. Deletion of p-test

K10

Asthma is an important anaesthetic consideration. It is unlikely that elective surgery would proceed in case of severe asthma, but it is not uncommon to be asked for assistance if a symptomatic asthma patient presents as an emergency. Asthma can be fatal even in previously well-controlled patients so, like many anaesthetic dangers, a well-rehearsed algorithm for dealing with problems is essential.

In asthma:
a. The major limitation of airflow in asthma is during the inspiratory phase
b. Hypercapnoea is a sign of reduced minute volume, but is not necessarily an indication for immediate intubation
c. Normocapnoea combined with hypoxia is indicative of adequate minute volume in the context of inadequate oxygen transfer
d. Oxygen should be given at high concentrations except if there is hypercapnoea
e. When using magnesium sulphate, large doses may be given and, if response is inadequate, infusion rates should be doubled

K11

A 24-year-old female has suffered substantial burns when her clothing caught fire after pouring petrol on a barbeque. On arrival in the emergency department, she is intubated to protect her airway. Secondary survey reveals extensive burns to her chest, thighs and circumferential burns to her arms. After initial fluid resuscitation, the surgeons ask to take her directly from the emergency department to theatre.

For what reason do the surgeons wish to take this patient to theatre?
a. Debride her burns
b. Perform escharotomies on her arms
c. Perform an immediate tracheostomy
d. Graft her thighs and arms
e. Establish a nasojejunal feeding tube

K12

You have been asked to anaesthetize an ex-premature baby, born at 32 weeks' gestation, for elective bilateral inguinal hernia repair. His corrected gestational age is 60 weeks and he weighs 3.5 kg. He was discharged home 24 weeks ago without ancillary oxygen and has been well in himself.

What would be your preferred anaesthetic technique?
a. Caudal block with sedation
b. General anaesthesia with 0.3 mg of intravenous morphine and intravenous infusion of paracetamol 22.5 mg
c. General anaesthesia with bilateral ilioinguinal blocks
d. General anaesthesia with caudal block
e. Spinal anaesthesia with sedation

K13

A 70-year-old male patient with postcentral stroke pain has been on increasing doses of oral morphine solution. He is now taking 180 mg per day. It is decided to switch his opioid medication to an alternative in order to achieve better analgesia.

Which would be an appropriate equipotent dose?
a. Oxycodone 360 mg po per day
b. Fentanyl 50 mcg/h patch every 72 hours
c. Tramadol 400 mg po per day
d. Methadone 300 mg po per day
e. Buprenorphine 20 mcg/h patch every 7 days

K14

You have admitted a patient with Burkitt's lymphoma to ICU from the haematology ward. He has been oliguric following his first dose of chemotherapy earlier today and his renal function has deteriorated significantly. A diagnosis of tumour lysis syndrome is suspected.

Which of the following is not used in the management of tumour lysis syndrome?
a. Forced alkaline diuresis
b. Allopurinol
c. Rasburicase

d. Renal replacement therapy
e. Dexamethasone

K15

You are due to anaesthetize a 68-year-old woman with ischaemic heart disease and poor exercise tolerance. She has an extensive breast lump, which the surgeon believes she can remove under local anaesthesia. The surgeon tells you she will require a total of 80 ml of solution to cover the area during surgery. You have to make up the solution.

Which of the following solutions would be appropriate for a 60-kg woman?
a. 18 ml of 2% lidocaine, 2.5 ml 1:1000 adrenaline, made up to 80 ml with 0.9% saline
b. 21 ml of 2% lidocaine, 0.4 ml 1:1000 adrenaline, made up to 80 ml with 0.9% saline
c. 9 ml of 2% lidocaine, 2.5 ml 1:1000 adrenaline, made up to 80 ml with 0.9% saline
d. 42 ml of 2% lidocaine, 0.4 ml 1:1000 adrenaline, made up to 80 ml with 0.9% saline
e. 6 ml of 2% lidocaine, 2.5 ml 1:1000 adrenaline, made up to 80 ml with 0.9% saline

K16

A 45-year-old haemophiliac presents for a femoral nailing following an RTA. His factor VIII concentration is 20% of normal and his haemoglobin is 100 g/l.

Which of the following statements is true?
a. Factor VIII levels should be raised to 50% of normal with fresh frozen plasma
b. Factor VIII levels should be raised using fresh whole blood
c. He should receive one unit of cryoprecipitate
d. Preoperative factor VIII levels should be 80% using factor VIII concentrate
e. Postoperative factor VIII levels should be maintained at 30% for 1 day with factor VIII concentrate

K17

In patients with liver disease undergoing surgery, a mortality risk can be estimated using the Child–Pugh classification.

Which one of the following is not included in Pugh's modification of Child's criteria?
a. Ascites
b. Grade of encephalopathy
c. Serum albumin
d. Activated partial thromboplastin time
e. Serum bilirubin

K18

A 36-year-old multigravida is undergoing Caesarean section following failed trial of forceps. Shortly after administration of prophylactic antibiotics, she complains of dyspnoea, and the surgeon complains of excessive bleeding from wound edges. There is wheeze on auscultation, you administer oxygen, but the patient becomes more restless, cyanosed and unresponsive.

The likely diagnosis is:
a. Amniotic fluid embolism
b. Massive pulmonary embolism
c. HELLP syndrome

d. Anaphylaxis
e. Acute asthma

K19

A 10-year-old child with a history of weight loss, polydipsia and polyuria is brought into the emergency department with a pulse of 120/min. She is found to be drowsy and uncommunicative. Her blood sugar is 22, pH 7.02 and ketones are present in her urine.

Which of the following statements is incorrect?
a. High-flow oxygen via a facemask should be administered
b. Intubation and ventilation may be required
c. A bolus of 10–30 ml/kg of 0.9% saline should be given
d. An actrapid infusion at 0.1 unit/kg per hour should be commenced
e. The acidosis needs to be treated with sodium bicarbonate

K20

The development of chronic pain is due in part to the sensitization of dorsal horn neurones.

Which of the following receptors is thought to play a central role in this process?
a. AMPA
b. GABA
c. Kainate
d. NMDA
e. TRPV1

K21

A 50-year-old female is admitted to the ICU from the Emergency Department with acute liver failure. She has taken an overdose of 50 grams of paracetamol 24 hours previously. She has been adequately fluid resuscitated since admission.

Which of the following criteria would make her a candidate for super-urgent liver transplantation?
a. Prothrombin time >100 seconds irrespective of the grade of encephalopathy
b. Age >40 years, prothrombin time >50 seconds and serum bilirubin >308 µmol/l
c. Prothrombin time >100 seconds and serum creatinine >301 µmol/l
d. Arterial pH < 7.3 and grade 3 or 4 encephalopathy
e. Arterial pH < 7.3 irrespective of grade of encephalopathy

K22

You are working on the obstetric unit and are called to see a 30-year-old primigravida with a BMI of 41. The patient is having regular contractions and the cervix is dilated to 4 cm. She is coping well on entonox currently, but asks you if, and when, you would advise siting an epidural.

Which would be the most appropriate response?
a. Advise that she has an epidural when she can no longer manage labour pain with entonox alone
b. Assess her airway and, if found to be difficult, advise early epidural insertion
c. Site iv access, explain the procedure and take consent, so that you are ready to place an epidural at short notice if required

217

d. Advise early epidural and iv access regardless of current pain level and airway assessment
e. Examine the patient's spine and judge potential for difficulty before deciding on the course of action

K23

An 8-day old baby, born at full term, had an antenatal diagnosis of congenital diaphragmatic hernia and required intubation and ventilation shortly after birth. You are anaesthetizing him for repair of the hernia. Shortly after the abdomen is closed, his blood pressure drops to 65/35 mmHg, heart rate falls from 145 to 90 bpm and oxygen saturations fall to 55%.

Which of the following is the least likely diagnosis?
a. Tension pneumothorax around the hypoplastic lung
b. Tension pneumothorax of the contralateral lung
c. Inferior vena cava compression
d. Increased abdominal pressure causing respiratory embarrassment
e. Pulmonary hypertension causing right-to-left shunt

K24

Following a rapid sequence induction for an emergency appendicectomy you notice that the patient feels difficult to ventilate and has developed a widespread urticarial rash. On auscultation, breaths sounds are equal bilaterally but there is widespread wheeze. The blood pressure is unrecordable, but there is a weak carotid pulse.

Which of the following is the most appropriate drug treatment?
a. Adrenaline 0.5 ml of 1 in 1000 im, hydrocortisone 50 mg
b. Adrenaline 0.5 ml of 1 in 10000 iv, hydrocortisone 200 mg
c. Adrenaline 0.5 ml of 1 in 1000 iv, hydrocortisone 50 mg
d. Adrenaline 0.5 ml of 1 in 1000 im, hydrocortisone 200 mg
e. Adrenaline 1.0 ml of 1 in 10000 iv, hydrocortisone 100 mg

K25

A phenytoin infusion extravasates from a peripheral cannula. You stop the infusion and disconnect the line from the cannula.

The next most appropriate action would be to:
a. Administer 1500 units hyaluronidase immediately through the cannula
b. Administer 200 mg hydrocortisone intravenously
c. Aspirate as much drug as possible from the cannula
d. Perform a stellate ganglion block
e. Refer to a plastic surgeon for urgent liposuction

K26

A 25-year-old woman in early labour at term complains of right calf pain. Of note, she had developed a deep vein thrombosis in her previous pregnancy.

Which of the following options is most accurate regarding the management of this patient?
a. A raised D-dimer result is useful when confirming a deep vein thrombosis
b. Low molecular weight heparin therapy may be continued through labour, until the start of the second stage

c. Regional anaesthesia should not be undertaken until at least 12 hours after the last dose of therapeutic LMWH
d. An epidural catheter should not be removed within 6 hours of a dose of LMWH
e. A thrombo-prophylactic dose of LMWH may be given 4 hours after Caesarean section

K27

Regarding pharmacological strategies used to protect kidneys perioperatively, which of the following statements is false?
a. Dopamine may increase renal perfusion pressure and improve urine output
b. Dopexamine, when used perioperatively for vascular patients, does not protect kidneys
c. Volatile anaesthetic agents may have a role to play in decreasing renal reperfusion injury
d. Cardiac surgical patients with early acute kidney injury, if treated with recombinant human atrial natriuretic peptide, may not progress to the severe form needing dialysis
e. Intravascular fluids along with prophylactic N-acetylcysteine have no role in the prevention of radiocontrast nephropathy

K28

The most common congenital cardiac lesion with an incidence of 35% is:
a. Ventricular septal defect
b. Atrial septal defect
c. Patent ductus arteriosus
d. Tetralogy of Fallot
e. Coarctation

K29

An 18-year-old man with small bowel obstruction is booked by the general surgeons for an urgent laparotomy. The patient has Duchenne's muscular dystrophy (DMD) and is confined to a wheelchair. He has a mild scoliosis and an FVC > 70% of that predicted.

Which of the following pieces of equipment would be most useful intraoperatively?
a. Intubating laryngeal mask airway
b. Transoesophageal echocardiography machine
c. Neuromuscular monitoring
d. Bispectral index monitor
e. 'Volatile-free' anaesthetic machine

K30

A 45-year-old woman is to undergo a laparotomy for the removal of an ileo-caecal tumour. She reports intermittent episodes of flushing, hypotension, dizziness and diarrhoea, especially when anxious. A 24-hour urine collection showed raised levels of 5-hydroxyindoleacetic acid.

Which of the following perioperative measures will be of most benefit?
a. Epidural infusion of local anaesthetic
b. Rapid sequence induction of anaesthesia (RSI)
c. Preoperative octreotide infusion
d. Transthoracic echocardiography
e. Intraoperative vasopressin infusion

Paper K – Answers

K1

Answer: d.

There are two types of stents: bare-metal stents (BMS) and drug-eluting stents (DES). Stent thrombosis is rare (~1%), most commonly occurring in the first month after insertion before re-endothelialization is complete. This may lead to MI or death, therefore patients with BMS are usually treated with clopidogrel for 6 weeks to allow for complete endothelial re-growth. In contrast, the anti-proliferative drugs released by DES delay endothelial growth, requiring treatment with clopidogrel for a minimum of 12 months. All patients with stents should continue to take low-dose aspirin for life.

Stopping clopidogrel during endothelial re-growth carries an estimated 30-fold increased risk of stent thrombosis. Invasive procedures increase this risk due to a prothrombotic state. The risk is reduced for BMS if surgery is performed >6 weeks after insertion. Timing of surgery after DES implantation is less clear, but is likely to be at least 12 months during which dual antiplatelet therapy (DAPT) must be maintained.

In the majority of surgical procedures, low-dose aspirin does not increase the severity of bleeding complications. General opinion is that clopidogrel will increase surgical bleeding and most practitioners recommend stopping it before elective surgery where possible. Both aspirin and clopidogrel inhibit platelet function irreversibly. The lifespan of a platelet is around 10 days; hence, restoration of normal platelet function in patients taking aspirin or clopidogrel takes 5–10 days.

Perioperatively, irreversible antiplatelet agents may be substituted with a reversible and short-acting anticoagulant and/or antiplatelet drug to offer thrombosis prophylaxis. There is little evidence for one regime over another. Examples include: unfractionated heparin (UFH), subcutaneous injection of low molecular weight heparin, non-steroidal anti-inflammatory drugs and GPIIb/IIIa inhibitors. If surgery cannot be delayed, a discussion regarding the risk of continuing DAPT vs. the risk of perioperative bleeding should be held between surgeon, anaesthetist, and cardiologist.

DeVile P, Foëx P. Antiplatelet drugs, coronary stents, and non-cardiac surgery. *Contin Educ Anaesth Crit Care Pain* 2010; **10** (6): 187–191

Practice Single Best Answer Questions for the Final FRCA, ed. Hozefa Ebrahim, Khalid Hasan, Mark Tindall, Michael Clarke and Natish Bindal. Published by Cambridge University Press. © Cambridge University Press 2013.

K2

Answer: d.

Gastric lavage and induced emesis are not routinely recommended as they have not been shown to be of benefit and can result in significant morbidity and mortality. Alkaline diuresis may be appropriate in salicylate toxicity, but not paracetamol. N-acetylcysteine is administered based on plasma paracetamol concentration, but initial treatment would be activated charcoal as it would be safe to administer in this situation and can reduce paracetamol absorption up to 2 hours' post ingestion.

Vaja R, McNicol L, and Sisley I. Anaesthesia for patients with liver disease. *Contin Educ Anaesth Crit Care Pain* 2010; **10** (1): 15–19

K3

Answer: d.

Cyanide is released from burning polyurethane foam. Upon inhalation, it inhibits cellular cytochrome oxidase, blocking the tricarboxylic acid cycle and stopping cellular respiration. Acute poisoning causes dizziness, headache, palpitations, breathlessness, drowsiness, coma, convulsions, pulmonary oedema and metabolic acidosis, all due to increasing hypoxia. These features would not be present at relatively low levels of carbon monoxide (<15%). The Health and Safety Executive no longer recommend a cyanide antidote, instead concentrating on supportive therapy, including maximizing oxygen delivery.

> 'HSE will no longer recommend the use of any antidote in the first aid treatment of cyanide poisoning and will not require employers to keep supplies. There is a great deal of anecdotal evidence of the value of oxygen and the experience of most occupational physicians is that the majority of victims of mild to moderate cyanide poisoning improve rapidly when treated with oxygen alone. HSE will in future advise that administration of oxygen is the most useful initial treatment for cyanide poisoning'.

Health and Safety Executive. Cyanide Poisoning – New Recommendations on First Aid Treatment. Health and Safety Executive, 2011

K4

Answer: c.

A range of approaches to the brachial plexus have been described; however, it is important that the anaesthetist chooses the most appropriate one depending on the patient and the intended surgery. The interscalene approach reliably blocks the shoulder and upper arm, but due to the position of the C8/T1 nerve roots the ulnar side of the arm is often not well covered. In such a case, a supplementary block of the ulnar nerve at the elbow can provide the necessary anaesthesia.

The commonest approach to the brachial plexus is via the axillary route. The complications associated with this route are fewer compared with other approaches. However, it is only really effective for surgery on the hand and forearm.

If the aim is anaesthesia of the entire arm, then the supraclavicular approach is usually the most effective in providing this. However, it is the technique with the highest incidence of pneumothorax. The most common technique is the subclavian approach described by Winnie.

Yentis S, Hirsch N, Smith G. *Anaesthesia and Intensive Care A–Z: An Encyclopaedia of Principles and Practice*, 4th edn, 2009. Edinburgh: Churchill Livingstone Elsevier

K5
Answer: a.

Neurolytic agents such as phenol and alcohol are indicated for use in cancer and peripheral vascular disease. They should be used with caution in other conditions. Local anaesthetics, with or without steroid, do not produce neurolysis. The most common neurolytic solutions are alcohol and phenol. Both sensory and motor nerve fibres are destroyed by phenol. However, at a concentration of 2%–3% motor nerve fibres are spared. As fibres can regenerate, these blocks are not permanent. Alcohol is more effective at destroying the nerve cell body and these blocks are more profound. In practice, however, 50%–100% alcohol is used. Local anaesthetics are often used as the diluents.

Rajesh AM, Swanepoel A. Sympathetic blocks. *Contin Educ Anaesth Crit Care Pain* 2010; 10(3): 88–92

K6
Answer: a.

The persistent failure of tubular function in chronic renal failure leads to the retention of potassium and urea, resulting in a raised anion gap, and a low bicarbonate level (acidosis). Conn's disease (hyperaldosteronism) results in hypernatraemia and hypokalaemia. Type 1 renal tubular acidosis (RTA) is a failure of the distal nephron to secrete acid, resulting in an inability to acidify the urine, and a tendency to normal anion gap acidaemia and hypokalaemia. Type 4 RTA is not due to tubular dysfunction, but a physiological reduction in proximal ammonia secretion, often due to hyperaldosteronism. There is a mild, normal anion gap, acidosis and hyperkalaemia. Analgesic nephropathy and antibiotics are the most common cause of acute interstitial nephritis, which may give rise to the aforementioned metabolic picture, but nephropathy is caused by paracetamol and other NSAIDs, not by opioid analgesics.

The anion gap is calculated by subtracting the sum of the major plasma anions (chloride and bicarbonate) from the sum of the major plasma cations (sodium and potassium). The value of the anion gap represents the unmeasured anions in the plasma.

$$([Na^+] + [K^+]) - ([Cl^-] + [HCO_3^-])$$

With normal plasma concentrations of these electrolytes, the normal anion gap is around 10–20 mmol/l, but quoted normal ranges vary and results must be interpreted according to local laboratory reference ranges. A metabolic acidosis with a raised anion gap suggests that an unmeasured anion is present, often lactic acid or a ketoacid. Bicarbonate is consumed as it buffers the acid, resulting in a decrease in the net anion concentration, and thus an increase in the value of the anion gap.

Causes of a raised anion gap metabolic acidosis are often referred to by the mnemonic MUDPILES:

M   Methanol
U   Uraemia (chronic renal failure)
D   Diabetic ketoacidosis
P   Propylene glycol
I   Infection, isoniazid, iron
L   Lactic acidosis
E   Ethylene glycol
S   Salicylates

K7

Answer: d.

Trimeprazine is a sedating antihistamine. Although popular in the past, it is less effective than midazolam. Ketamine has anxiolytic and sedative properties and is rapidly absorbed after oral administration. However, it is associated with hypersalivation, hallucinations and emergence phenomena, which may be problematic. Midazolam is the most commonly used sedative premedicant in UK paediatric practice. 0.5 mg/kg po produces excellent anxiolysis and reduces post-operative behavioural disturbances. Sedative effects are seen within 5–10 minutes, peak effect occurs within 20–30 minutes and the effect is waning at 45 minutes.

Intranasal administration of 0.2 mg/kg requires less patient cooperation and has a rapid effect. If parenteral administration is used, the dose is 0.1–0.2 mg/kg.

Tan L, Meakin GH. Anaesthesia for the uncooperative child. *Contin Educ Anaesth Crit Care Pain* 2010; **10** (2): 48–52

K8

Answer: c.

Epidural steroid injections must be performed under X-ray screening with non-ionic, low osmolar (myelogram) contrast. In the absence of X-ray screening only 50% of epidural steroid injections are in the epidural space. Of the 50% in the epidural space only half (i.e. 25% of the total) are at the correct level.

Ultrasound has been used to detect the spinal column but not accurate placement in the epidural space. Review of the preoperative CT scan is useful but real-time positioning is crucial. Peripheral nerve stimulation has been used in epidural placement but lacks the accuracy of X-ray screening.

Collighan N, Gupta S. Epidural steroids. *Contin Educ Anaesth Crit Care Pain* 2010; **10**(1): 1–5

K9

Answer: d.

Delirium is a common, under-estimated problem in ICU patients that is multi-factorial in origin. The mainstay of treatment is to minimize and correct risk factors along with regular screening of patients.

The Confusion Assessment Method for ICU (CAM-ICU) is derived from the confusion assessment method. It has a high sensitivity (93%–100%) and specificity (89%–100%). It is a simple test that can be performed by all ICU staff and is currently the only validated delirium tool for patients requiring ventilatory support. It requires an initial assessment of the level of consciousness or arousal by using a standard sedation score, e.g. Richmond Agitation Sedation Scale (RASS) and those patients scoring −3 or greater (on a scale of −5 to +4) can then be further assessed for delirium. The assessor asks the patient to squeeze their hand on the letter A and reads out ten letters, four of which are A. This will pick up evidence of inattention. Disorganized thinking is detected by asking the patient four simple yes/no questions and then issuing a simple command.

The Intensive Care Delirium Screening Checklist (ICDSC) is a useful screening tool, but gives a relatively high false-positive rate and is recommended only as a screening rather than as a diagnostic tool. The Ramsay scale was the first scale to be defined for sedated patients and is a test of reusability rather than delirium. The deletion of p-test is a tool used in the recovery room to assess cognitive/psychomotor function.

King J, Gratrix A. Delirium in intensive care. *Contin Educ Anaesth Crit Care Pain* 2009; **9**(5): 144–147

Ely EW, Inouye SK, Bernard GR *et al*. Delirium in mechanically ventilated patients: validity and reliability of the confusion assessment method for the intensive care unit. *J Am Med Assoc* 2001; **286**: 2703–2710

K10

Answer: b.

The major limitation of airflow in asthma is in the expiratory phase. This gives rise to the characteristic wheeze of asthma. Beware, though, of the silent chest as this may indicate insufficient airflow to generate audible wheeze.

Hypercapnoea is a sign of reduced minute volume requiring treatment, but is not necessarily dangerous in itself (hypoxia being much more dangerous). Patients with acute severe asthma are often hypocapnoeic as they are hyperventilating. Normocapnoea may be due either to resolution of the problem and normalization of blood gases or to a decrease in minute volume due to worsening of the condition. Be alert to the possibility that CO_2 in the normal range may not be a good sign. Hypercapnoea is not necessarily an indication for intubation, but is an ominous sign that should prompt re-evaluation of the situation at the very least. The safety of permissive hypercapnoea is well established and it is known that striving for normocapnoea may cause significant morbidity.

Hypoxia kills asthmatic patients. The Royal College of Anaesthetists emphasizes this year after year when examination candidates do not mention oxygen in their treatment algorithms. Hypercapnoea in these patients does not represent 'CO$_2$ retaining' in the same way as it might in COPD patients. If the patient is hypoxic, they are in need of oxygen, whatever their P_aCO_2 might be.

Magnesium sulphate is a useful treatment for bronchospasm, but it carries risks. Follow the British Thoracic Society guidelines to ensure optimal treatment.

Stanley D, Tunnicliffe B. Management of life threatening asthma in adults. *Contin Educ Anaesth Crit Care Pain* 2003; **8**(3): 95–99

Tuxen D, Leong T. The effects of ventilatory pattern on hyperinflation, airway pressures, and circulation in mechanical ventilation of patients with severe air-flow obstruction. *Am Rev Respir Dis* 1987; **142**: 872–879

K11

Answer: b.

There are few indications to take a burns patient directly to theatre. Debridement of burns is often performed between 1 and 3 days post burn to allow for complete resuscitation and evaluation of the burn areas. This interval also allows the full extent of cellular damage to become evident; debriding and grafting on to tissue that may ultimately be non-viable will simply waste donor site tissue. Blood flow to a burn peaks between 5–9 days and this represents the maximal risk for blood loss. Escharotomies are essential in circumferential burns, which may quickly contract and compromise distal blood supply to a limb. Emergency tracheostomy may be necessary in case of airway involvement, but this patient is already intubated. Early feeding is vital for burns nutrition, but nasogastric feeding is usually sufficient in the early care of the burns patient.

Herndon D (ed.). *Total Burn Care*, 3rd edn, 2007. Saunders

K12

Answer: d.

This baby does not have a strong indication for performing the operation under a purely regional or local technique. Since he went home at 36 weeks' gestational age, it is unlikely that he required invasive ventilatory support as a neonate. He has been well since he was discharged. In sick babies, the operation can be done under local or regional technique alone. It is preferable to avoid opioids in ex-premature infants due to the increased risk of apnoeic episodes.

The intravenous paracetamol dosage should be 7.5 mg/kg for babies that are less than 10 kg, maximum daily dose of less than 60 mg/kg per 24 hours.

It is important to ensure the total dosage required for bilateral field blocks does not exceed the safety limit. The duration of the spinal may not be sufficient for bilateral hernia repairs.

MHRA Drug Safety Update (July 2010). *Drug Safety Advice: Intravenous Paracetamol (Perfalgan): Risk of Accidental Overdose, Especially in Infants and Neonates.* **3**, (12, 2.)

K13

Answer: b.

The many forms of opioid preparations available may confuse the uninitiated. The fact remains that morphine sulphate (MS) is the gold-standard opioid and that there is no evidence to favour one specific opioid over another. Modified or sustained-release preparations are usually preferable to immediate-release preparations. Often, in pain conditions which are difficult to treat, such as post-central stroke pain, opioids can be switched in an attempt to achieve better analgesic control. There isn't always an obvious reason why one opioid should suit a patient more than another, and it can often be trial and error. Patients on doses greater than 180 mg oral morphine sulphate per day (or equivalent) should be managed by specialists in secondary care. Approximate equivalent doses of opioids mentioned in the question are below:

a. Oral MS to oral oxycodone – ratio 2:1
b. Oral MS to transdermal fentanyl – total 24-hour oral MS dose / 3.6 = transdermal fentanyl patch strength (in mcg/h)
c. Oral MS to oral tramadol – ratio 1: 0.1
d. Oral MS (90–300 mg) to oral methadone – ratio 8:1 (variable; ratio increases as MS dose increases)
e. Oral MS to buprenorphine – total 24-hour oral MS dose/1.7 = transdermal buprenorphine patch strength (in mcg/h)

British Pain Society Guidelines *Opioids for Persistent Pain: Good Practice* 2010. Source: http://www.britishpainsociety.org/pub_professional.htm

Coupe MH, Stannard C. Opioids in persistent non-cancer pain. *Contin Educ Anaesth Crit Care Pain* 2007; 7(3):100–103

K14

Answer: e.

Tumour lysis syndrome (TLS) is most commonly associated with treatment of the acute leukaemias and high-grade lymphomas, especially Burkitt's lymphoma. In certain rare cases, it can happen spontaneously, but most commonly occurs after treatment with chemotherapy (and occasionally with single-therapy dexamethasone treatment). TLS results in potentially life-threatening hyperkalaemia, renal failure and acidosis. Serum hyperphosphataemia and hypocalcaemia may also be present along with increased serum and urine uric acid. Management includes: aggressive fluid hydration and hyperkalaemia treatment, which may include renal replacement therapy, combined with the administration of rasburicase (a recombinant urate oxidase enzyme). Forced alkaline diuresis has previously been advocated, but its use is declining due to variable efficacy, especially where renal function is already compromised, and where there are complications such as fluid overload. Where TLS is likely to occur, close monitoring of renal function, calcium, phosphate and urate levels are required (e.g. 2, 4 and 8h after starting chemotherapy). Allopurinol or rasburicase are commonly used as prophylaxis where there is a high tumour load, and thus increased risk of TLS. Where rasburicase is used, allopurinol should be withheld.

Beed M, Levitt M, Bokhari SW. Intensive care management of patients with haematological malignancy. *Contin Educ Anaesth Crit Care Pain* 2009; 9(4): 167–171

K15

Answer: b.

The maximum safe dose of lidocaine is 3 mg/kg. With adrenaline, this increases to 7 mg/kg. In this volume, the resulting lidocaine solution would be 0.5%. The surgeon needs to know that this is a relatively weak solution of lidocaine, and this needs to be taken into consideration when performing surgery. To make a solution of 1:200 000 adrenaline, 0.4 ml of 1:1000 needs to be added to 80 ml of saline. In a patient with ischaemic heart disease, it would be unwise to use an adrenaline solution of greater than 1:200 000 concentration.

K16

Answer: d.

Haemophilia is an X-linked congenital bleeding disorder. It has a frequency of approximately one in 10000 births. A deficiency of coagulation factor VIII is known as haemophilia A and represents 80%–85% of haemophiliacs. Haemophilia B is caused by a deficiency in factor IX.

The following table correlates clotting factor level with the severity of bleeding:

Severity	Clotting factor level % activity (IU/ml)	Bleeding
Severe	1% (<0.011)	Spontaneous bleeding, mainly joints and muscles
Moderate	1%–5% (0.01–0.05)	Occasional spontaneous bleeding. Severe bleeding with trauma, surgery
Mild	5%–40% (0.05–0.40)	Severe bleeding with trauma or surgery

Although FFP, cryoprecipitate and DDAVP can be used to raise factor VIII levels, these are no longer used routinely. It is recommended that, for major surgery, the factor levels should be 80%–100% preoperatively and then maintained at high levels for several days postoperatively.

World Federation of Hemophilia. *Guidelines for the Management of Hemophilia*, 2005. Montreal, Canada

K17

Answer: d.

Child–Pugh classification of severity of liver disease

Modified Child–Pugh classification of severity of liver disease according to the degree of ascites, the plasma concentrations of bilirubin and albumin, the prothrombin time and the degree of encephalopathy

Parameter	Points assigned		
	1	2	3
Ascites	Absent	Slight	Moderate
Bilirubin, mg/dl	≤2	2–3	>3
Albumin, g/dl	>3.5	2.8–3.5	<2.8
Prothrombin time			
Seconds over control	1–3	4–6	>6
INR	<1.8	1.8–2.3	>2.3
Encephalopathy	None	Grade 1–2	Grade 3–4

A total score of 5–6 is considered grade A (well-compensated disease); 7–9 is grade B (significant functional compromise); and 10–15 is grade C (decompensated disease). These grades correlate with 1- and 2-year patient survival.

Vaja R, McNicol L, Sisley I. Anaesthesia for patients with liver disease. *Contin Educ Anaesth Crit Care Pain* 2010; **10**(1): 15–19

K18

Answer: a.

This patient has suffered an amniotic fluid embolism. This is a rare event resulting from amniotic fluid entering the mother's bloodstream via the placental bed of the uterus. This is an obstetric and anaesthetic emergency with anaphylactic and embolic features. This reaction results in cardiorespiratory collapse and coagulopathy.

Risk factors for developing amniotic fluid embolism include:

- Increased maternal age
- Augmented labour
- Caesarean section
- Instrumental delivery
- Polyhydramnios
- Uterine rupture
- Placental abruption

Gist RS, Stafford IP, Leibowits AB *et al*. Amniotic fluid embolism. *Anaesth Analg* 2009; **108**(5): 1599–1602

K19

Answer: e.

She has presented with diabetic ketoacidosis (DKA). Children can die from DKA as a result of cerebral oedema, hypokalaemia and aspiration pneumonia. As with all emergencies, an assessment of airway, breathing and circulation is initially performed. It is important to weigh the child as soon as possible to guide fluid replacement and drug dosage. Bicarbonate is rarely indicated; however, may be considered when the pH < 6.9 and circulatory failure is evident. Its purpose is to improve cardiac contractility in severe shock, but may cause paradoxical cellular acidosis.

Edge, J. *Guidelines for the Management of Diabetic Ketoacidosis*. British Society of Paediatric Endocrinology and Diabetes, 2009

K20

Answer: d.

Pain signals that persist beyond the acute stage are not fully understood, but involve several linked mechanisms.

Following an injury, nerves can become sensitized and discharge at lowered thresholds. C-fibres can develop new adrenergic receptors; this may go some way to explaining the mechanism of sympathetically mediated pain. Damaged nerves can form dysfunctional sodium channels, which produce ectopic discharges.

Inflammatory mediators such as substance P and prostaglandins are released from damaged nerves. These can activate surrounding nociceptors. Following a peripheral nerve injury, changes within the central nervous system (CNS) can persist. This plasticity within the CNS is important in the development of chronic pain states. Repetitive stimulation of C-fibres can result in 'wind-up', where the rate of firing of dorsal horn cells will increase with the duration of the stimulus. Repetitive episodes of wind-up may precipitate 'long-term potentiation'. Long-term potentiation is defined as a long-lasting increase in synaptic activity. The NMDA receptor is believed to play an important role in these sensitization processes.

Alterations in the descending pathways from the brainstem and higher centres will also play a role in the development of chronic pain states. This is complex, but will involve the areas involved in the sensory-discriminative aspects of pain such as intensity and location, as in well as in centres involved in the affective-cognitive aspects of pain including anxiety, emotion and memory.

Harvey V, Dickenson A. Neurobiology of pain, in Stannard C, Kalso E, Ballantyne J (eds). *Evidence-based Chronic Pain Management*, 2010. Blackwell Publishing

K21

Answer: e.

The King's College Hospital Criteria are used to guide the need for transplantation in fulminant hepatic failure.

For paracetamol-induced liver failure, the following criteria indicate need for liver transplantation:

Arterial pH <7.3 (irrespective of the grade of encephalopathy)

or

Grade III or IV encephalopathy, *and*
Prothrombin time >100 seconds, *and*
Serum creatinine >3.4 mg/dl (301 μmol/l)

For all other causes of fulminant hepatic failure, the following criteria are used:

Prothrombin time >100 seconds (irrespective of the grade of encephalopathy)

or

Any three of the following variables (irrespective of the grade of encephalopathy)

1. Age <10 years or >40 years
2. Etiology: non-A, non-B hepatitis, halothane hepatitis, idiosyncratic drug reactions
3. Duration of jaundice before onset of encephalopathy >7 days
4. Prothrombin time >50 seconds
5. Serum bilirubin >18 mg/dl (308 μmol/l)

O'Grady JG, Graeme JM, Hayllar KM, Williams R. Early indicators of prognosis in fulminant hepatic failure. *Gastroenterology* 1989; **97**: 439–445

K22

Answer: d.

Morbidly obese patients are at high risk of difficult iv access, difficult epidural placement, difficult airway and postpartum haemorrhage.

A good, working epidural can improve cardiorespiratory parameters, give excellent labour analgesia and potentially obviate the need for intubation in the situation of an emergency Caesarean section.

However, technical procedures in the obese can be more challenging. It would be prudent to site an epidural as early as possible in such patients, when they are relatively less distressed and more able to keep still. This is also the time to have a more meaningful discussion about the risks and benefits of epidural anaesthesia, both in general, and more specifically for this patient.

Care of obese and morbidly obese parturients is becoming increasingly relevant. They pose many significant clinical problems and benefit from intensive, multi-disciplinary team care. The Royal College of Obstetricians and Gynaecologists has recently published a guideline on the care of such patients.

Pierson R, Alexander H, Calthorpe N. Obstetric anaesthesia and obesity. *Curr Wom Hlth Rev* 2011; 7(1): 94–100

CMACE/RCOG Joint Guideline: Management of women with obesity in pregnancy: online. Available at: http://www.rcog.org.uk/womens-health/clinical-guidance/management-women-obesity-pregnancy. Accessed 14.02.2012

K23

Answer: a.

Congenital diaphragmatic hernia (CDH) is associated with hypoplasia of the ipsilateral lung (which will also have abnormal pulmonary vasculature) and pulmonary hypertension. There may also be hypoplasia of the contralateral lung. CDH is associated with other abnormalities including:

- Cardiovascular (ASD/VSD, coarctation of aorta, tetralogy of Fallot)
- Central nervous system (spina bifida, hydrocephalus)
- Other gastrointestinal (malrotation or atresia)
- Genitourinary (hypospadias)

Clinical features of congenital diaphragmatic hernia include a scaphoid abdomen (due to lack of contents), barrel chest and presence of bowel sounds in the chest and shifted heart sounds. A chest X-ray will confirm diagnosis showing intrathoracic bowel loops (and possibly liver/spleen), and mediastinal shift.

The neonate should be stabilized with medical management preoperatively. Surgical repair of the hernia will not cause immediate restitution of the respiratory symptoms and the neonate remains at risk of pulmonary hypertension.

Intraoperatively, any sudden deterioration in cardiorespiratory status is suggestive of tension pneumothorax. The ipsilateral lung is hypoplastic and has very high inflation pressures and there should not be attempts to expand it. Any such attempts can easily result in contralateral tension pneumothorax (due to rupture of the normal alveoli), necessitating prompt decompression and insertion of a chest drain. Postoperatively, the surgeons will usually have inserted a chest drain on the operative side, so postoperative tension pneumothorax on this side is unlikely.

Repair of the hernia clearly involves returning abdominal contents to an under-developed abdominal cavity, which may not be able to accommodate the additional contents and results in higher intra-abdominal pressures. This may cause caval compression compromising venous return to the heart and hypotension with potential cardiovascular collapse. The increase in abdominal pressures can also cause respiratory embarrassment and atelectasis, which may result in high airway pressures and difficulty in ventilation. Neonatal pulmonary vasculature remains muscular, since it had accommodated the fetal systemic pressures. It retains sensitivity to vasoconstrictor effects such as hypoxia, hypothermia and acidosis. Persistent postoperative hypoxia suggests persistent pulmonary hypertension with right-to-left shunting.

Yao F, Fontes ML, Malhotra V. *Yao and Artusio's Anesthesiology: Problem-orientated Patient Management*, 6th edn, 2008. Philidephia: Lippincott Williams & Wilkins, 115–129

K24
Answer: b.

The incidence of anaphylactic reaction has been estimated at a rate of 1:10000 to 1:20000 anaesthetics. It is a life-threatening emergency and treatment must be immediate. Death usually occurs from asphyxiation or irreversible circulatory shock.

Adrenaline is the mainstay treatment with initially 50–100 mcg intravenously (0.5–1.0 ml of 1 in 10000) being recommended for adults by the AAGBI. This is slightly different from ALS guidelines which recommend im adrenaline. Repeat doses may be required if there is severe hypotension or bronchospasm. Secondary treatment can include corticosteroids, antihistamines and bronchodilators; however, these are of secondary importance to adrenaline.

AAGBI Suspected anaphylactic reactions associated with anaesthesia. *Anaesthesia* 2009; **64**: 199–211

K25
Answer: c.

Prompt appropriate management will minimize subsequent injury. The early management is stopping administration and aspiration to reduce the amount of drug present. For most extravasation injuries, treatment is aimed at reducing drug concentration at the site. Other treatments include limb elevation to promote venous drainage and warm compresses for vasodilatation – which increases drug reabsorption and distribution.

The other options all fall under secondary management and include:

- Saline washout
- Liposuction
- Steroids
- Hyaluronidase
- Phentolamine
- Regional sympathetic block

Lake C, Beecroft CL. Extravasation injuries and accidental intra-arterial injection. *Contin Educ Anaesth Crit Care Pain* 2010; **10**(4): 109–113

K26

Answer: e.

D-dimers can be elevated in pregnancy due to physiological changes in the coagulation system. LMWH should be stopped once the woman is in established labour, or thinks that she is in labour. In women on a therapeutic regimen of LMWH, regional techniques should not be used for at least 24 hours after the last dose of LMWH. Epidural catheters should not be removed until 12 hours after the last dose of LMWH. There is some conflicting advice in the RCOG guidelines regarding the time interval between lower segment Caesarean section with regional technique and administration of LMWH; however, the consensus is that 4 hours is a safe interval.

Nelson-Piercy C, MacCallum P, Mackillop L. *Reducing the Risk of Thrombosis and Embolism During Pregnancy and the Puerperium*, 2009. London: Royal College of Obstetricians and Gynaecologists

Greer IA, Thomson AJ. *The Acute Management of Thrombosis and Embolism during Pregnancy and the Puerperium*, 2010. London: Royal College of Obstetricians and Gynaecologists.

K27

Answer: e.

The style of this question is atypical for RCoA SBAs; however, it contains important learning points.

Dopamine is a catecholamine, which acts not only on the dopamine receptors but also on α- and β-receptors of the sympathetic nervous system, increasing cardiac output and the renal perfusion pressure. Dopamine receptors present in the renal system cause vasodilatation, which increases the renal blood flow. A combined effect of dopamine on the sympathetic and dopamine receptors leads to an improved urine output. Evidence does not support the use of low-dose dopamine for renal protection as it does not prevent renal failure or the need for dialysis, nor does it affect mortality. Dopexamine is a synthetic compound with similar effects to dopamine and like dopamine has not shown promising results in renal protection. Volatile anaesthetic agents have been shown to encourage preconditioning, a protective response, which may be responsible for reducing renal ischemic-reperfusion injury. Natriuretic peptides increase glomerular perfusion pressure and filtration by causing natriuresis. This effect is currently being investigated, though there is insufficient evidence supporting its use to prevent dialysis in patients with acute kidney injury. The use of antioxidant *N*-acetylcysteine (NAC) for prevention of renal injury due to contrast medium has been supported by the literature so far, although recent trials in cardiac and vascular surgery patients have shown conflicting results.

Webb ST, Allen JSD. Perioperative renal protection. *Contin Educ Anaesth Crit Care Pain* 2008; 8(5): 176–180

K28

Answer: a.

Mean per million:

| VSD 3570 |
| ASD 941 |
| PDA 799 |
| TOF 421 |
| Coarctation 409 |

Hoffman, JI, Kaplan, S. The incidence of congenital heart disease. *J Am Coll Cardiol* 2002; **39** (2): 1890–1900

K29

Answer: c.

The use of muscle relaxants in the sex-linked dystrophies is problematic. Depolarizing muscle relaxants are contra-indicated due to possible hyperkalaemia. Non-depolarizing muscle relaxants demonstrate a prolonged time to onset and prolonged duration of action; neuromuscular monitoring is therefore mandated.

Total intravenous anaesthesia is becoming the standard anaesthetic technique for patients with muscular dystrophy. A malignant hyperthermia-like phenomenon has been reported in these patients; this has been termed anaesthesia-related rhabdomyolysis (AIR).

Patients with muscular dystrophy would benefit from preoperative echocardiography and cardiology referral if there is developing heart failure, but intraoperative echocardiography is not required.

There is an increased incidence of difficult intubation, but this could be managed in a variety of ways.

Birnkrant DJ, Panitch HB, Benditt JO *et al*. American College of Chest Physicians Consensus Statement on the respiratory and related management of patients with Duchenne muscular dystrophy undergoing anesthesia or sedation. *Chest* 2007; **132**: 1977–1986

Hayes J, Veyckemans F, Bissonnette B. Duchenne muscular dystrophy: an old anesthesia problem revisited. *Paediatr Anesth* 2008; **18**: 100–106

K30

Answer: c.

This patient is to undergo resection of a carcinoid tumour. The symptoms that she reports are suggestive of the release of vasoactive peptides – this is the carcinoid syndrome. Crises can be triggered by emotional stress, pain, hypercapnoea, hypothermia, hypotension (through catecholamine release), histamine-releasing medication and hypertension (through the release of bradykinin). Low-dose epidural has been used successfully without triggering carcinoid crisis, a low-dose infusion should be used to avoid precipitating hypotension. Epidural anaesthesia will provide excellent intraoperative analgesia in addition. Morphine has been used, but may cause release of histamine.

In certain circumstances there may be a role for RSI. Preoperative investigations should include echocardiography to evaluate right-sided cardiac disease. Some vasopressors may cause the release of vasoactive peptides due to activation of the autonomic nervous system. Therefore, vasopressin may be a better choice.

Of paramount importance is the minimization of tumour secretory activity. Octreotide acts to suppress vasoactive mediator release. Its side effects include QT prolongation, bradycardia and conduction defects.

Powell B, Al Mukhtar A, Mills GH. Carcinoid: the disease and its implications for anaesthesia. *Contin Educ Anaesth Crit Care Pain* 2011; **11**: 9–13

Index

(Entries in bold are found in the answer sections; entries not in bold are found in the questions.)

Printed in the United States
By Bookmasters